P9-ECI-172

ALPHABET BLESSINGS

ALPHABET BLESSINGS

▼

Conceiving with In Vitro Fertilization

Jenifer A. Cotter, D.O.

iUniverse, Inc.
New York Lincoln Shanghai

Library Resource Center
Renton Technical College
3000 N.E. 4th St.
Renton, WA 98056

Alphabet Blessings
Conceiving with In Vitro Fertilization

Copyright © 2006 by Jenifer A. Cotter, D.O.

All rights reserved. No part of this book may be used or reproduced by any means, graphic, electronic, or mechanical, including photocopying, recording, taping or by any information storage retrieval system without the written permission of the publisher except in the case of brief quotations embodied in critical articles and reviews.

iUniverse books may be ordered through booksellers or by contacting:

iUniverse
2021 Pine Lake Road, Suite 100
Lincoln, NE 68512
www.iuniverse.com
1-800-Authors (1-800-288-4677)

ISBN-13: 978-0-595-39524-8 (pbk)
ISBN-13: 978-0-595-83923-0 (ebk)
ISBN-10: 0-595-39524-4 (pbk)
ISBN-10: 0-595-83923-1 (ebk)

Printed in the United States of America

618.1780599 COTTER 2006

Cotter, Jenifer A.

Alphabet blessings

Disclaimer

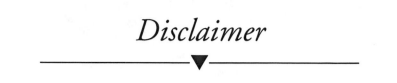

The content of this book is intended for educational and support purposes only. Nothing contained within this book is intended to be instructional for medical diagnosis or treatment.

Although the author has made a conscientious effort to provide high quality information, the author disclaims any implied guarantee about the accuracy, completeness, timeliness or relevance of any information contained herein.

The information in this book should not be relied on to suggest a course of treatment for a particular individual, and it should not be used in place of a visit, call, consultation or the advice of a physician or other healthcare provider. The reader should not disregard or postpone seeking medical advice from a physician or any other healthcare provider because of something contained in this book.

The author accepts no responsibility for actions taken by individuals in response to what they have read on these pages or on Web sites that have been provided for reference. Always check online sources of information for reliability and timeliness of content as indicated by author information and date of last site revision.

The information contained within this book is compiled from a variety of sources including medical journals, medical Web sites, conversations with medical colleagues, conversations with infertility couples and personal experience.

for my beautiful son
and loving husband

I hope my achievements in life shall be these—
that I will have fought for what was right and fair,
that I will have risked for that which mattered,
that I will have given help to those who were in need…
that I will have left the earth a better place for what
I've done and for who I've been.

C. Hoppe

Table of Contents

▼

Acknowledgments

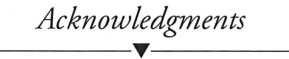

Reaching out to other infertile couples has been one of the most rewarding endeavors of my life. I have learned so much from some pretty amazing people and would like to take a moment to thank them.

At a time when I had all but lost faith in the medical community, Dr. Randy Morris offered his hand with sincerity and a smile. I can never thank you enough, Randy, for your amazing expertise in the field of ART, for your gentle care and most importantly, for the gift of my son.

I also owe a special thank you to Dr. Richard Barton for introducing me to Dr. Morris and for Dr. Barton's wonderful care throughout my pregnancy. Thank you, Rich, for helping Nicholas enter this world and for allowing me to spend so much time with him those first few weeks of life.

Words can never fully express my gratitude to all my friends and the families of the infertility community. You have all touched my life in such a positive way. For all the support I may have given you, you have given me so much more in return. A heartfelt thank you to all the members of my support group for making it such a success and such a haven for other infertility couples; to everyone who shared so much with me and entrusted me with their deepest thoughts and desires; and to everyone who encouraged me to follow my dream of writing this book.

Above all, I want to thank my family for their love and support through my days of trying to conceive and through the many ups and downs I have experienced while trying to find my path in this world. Thank you to my parents and sister for their love and devotion to Nicholas and to my nephew for taking Nick under his wing as though he were his little brother. Extra thanks to you, Mom, for contributing your heartfelt thoughts to my book and for all the nights you got almost no sleep so that I could have a much-needed new mom break! Thank you to my husband, Jeff, for supporting me while I pursued my passions, for devoting so much of himself to me while I was pregnant and for always believing in me, even when I didn't. I love you more each day, Jeff. You are forever and always my soul mate and an amazing father. And although he is yet too young to know my words of gratitude, I thank my son Nicholas for bringing me to a higher level in my life and for reminding me each day how blessed I am to know the joy of motherhood and the joy of raising such an amazing little boy. Nicholas, you are my everything. I love you.

Introduction

▼

Much like my journey to motherhood, my journey to publishing has been challenging. Four years ago, when I first put pen to paper, it seemed a simple undertaking: share my story, express my thoughts, offer my support to those still struggling. Yet this endeavor has been anything but simple. The greatest challenge for me hasn't been writing a book full of sound information. It hasn't been opening up and sharing some of the most personal and intimate moments of my life. Rather, the greatest challenge in writing this book has been conveying the positive aspects and beauty often hidden behind the otherwise technical and intrusive medical process of in vitro. Great time and energy has been dedicated to developing the book's tone and underlying message of hope, possibility, strength, and pride so that every reader walks away feeling inspired and empowered, ready to face all the challenges of infertility that might lie ahead.

I have been asked how I came to choose the title for this book. To me, *Alphabet Blessings* embraces the positive side of assisted conception and reaffirms the beauty of conceiving with in vitro fertilization. When you travel along the path of assisted conception, you find yourself swimming in a sea of letters: IVF, FET, ER, ET. At the end of that same path you may very well find a blessing, a tiny baby to call your own. I feel it is an uplifting title for this book and a wonderful way to describe the beautiful babies born each year with the help of in vitro fertilization. Much better than test tube babies, wouldn't you agree?

So, what will you find in this book? *Alphabet Blessings* truly is a well-balanced blend of my personal struggle with (and triumph over) infertility and the medical details of an in vitro fertilization cycle. More than anything, I want this book to feel personal. I have included entries from my personal IVF journal, comments from my husband and mother, embarrassing moments, and photos of my family. It's my way of inviting you into my life; a life I never thought I would experience and one I hope every couple comes to know themselves.

My infertility/IVF support efforts over the past six years have taught me that couples want more than a friendly shoulder or reassuring voice. Couples want and need information. During my infertility support endeavors, I have quickly learned that each couple is quite different when it comes to absorbing information. First, everyone learns differently. Some couples want to read medically-based information while others are seeking a personal story they can relate to. For every couple that wants to read a full article there is another couple who wishes to just see the highlights and key points of a topic.

Second, each couple is at a different emotional state. This is largely influenced by their journey to parenthood thus far. Newbies tend to be much more open and eager while veterans tend to be more cautious and reserved. Some couples are too fragile to read success stories while some eagerly search for fellow IVFers who have been blessed with their miracle babies.

Third, each couple hopes to achieve a different level of expertise regarding IVF. Some couples are seeking a general guide and don't wish to know the "why" but rather prefer to focus on the phase-by-phase breakdown of a cycle. Other couples are seeking detailed information and wish to learn why their physician is ordering certain tests or choosing a particular medication. These couples also want to know specific ways they can positively contribute to their IVF cycle.

This book strives to speak to every infertile couple regardless of their background or experience level. My personal story has been clearly separated from the medically oriented portions of this book, allowing each reader to choose which section they'd like to read. My personal story has been broken down into our struggle with infertility, our in vitro fertilization cycle and our pregnancy, so anyone not wishing to read about our pregnancy can skip that section. If you feel emotionally fragile and find it difficult to see baby pictures, please be forewarned that our personal story includes images of my pregnant belly and my son as a baby in the pregnancy chapter.

The second section of this book details life as an infertile couple and the phases of an in vitro cycle. Detailed medical information is contained in each of the chapters outlining the stages of IVF and in the chapter about factors affecting cycle outcome. Helpful hints and inspirational quotes are scattered throughout these chapters as well. Each chapter ends with a general overview to reiterate the key points in layman terms. If at anytime the terminology sounds confusing, simply flip to the glossary (alphabet soup and learn the lingo sections) at the back of the book for clarification. There is a tremendous amount of information to absorb and the terminology can be daunting. Almost every IVF couple feels somewhat overwhelmed when first beginning this journey but there is an incredible sense of empowerment to be gained through knowledge, so don't give up if you stumble through some of the medical sections your first time.

My greatest wish is that you never feel you must face this journey alone. Each couple may take away something different from this book, but every couple should feel positive for the path they have chosen. It is a scary and often twisted path and there is no guarantee about what lies at the end of the journey. Never doubt yourself and never lose sight of the possibilities which lie before you. Share what you learn from this book and reach out to others as I have reached out to you. If only one person smiles, if only one person feels inspired, if only one person finds strength in my words, then the book is so very worthwhile. Together we can make the journey easier and together we can show the world the beauty of assisted conception.

Preface

▼

In August 2000, my husband and I embarked on a journey unlike any other we had ever taken. We walked into a reproductive endocrinologist's office with aspirations of becoming parents. Little did we know just how exhausting our journey would be. Conception for most couples was a moment of passion, an act of love, a creation of one from two. But we were no ordinary couple. We were an infertility couple.

As we sat listening to our physician outline the procedure, the risks, the potential complications, and the uncertain outcome of in vitro fertilization, we realized that an incredible challenge lay before us. We would have to be ready to endure pain, stress and possible heartache. And we would need to risk our health and finances for the chance to hear those precious words, "Mommy" and "Daddy." I spent many restless nights wondering if we would overcome the odds or if we would also fall victim to the disheartening failure statistics.

One morning I stood looking in the mirror, pillow under my shirt doing what every woman battling infertility has done, trying to picture myself pregnant. I was tired of feeling like a prisoner to my menstrual cycle, tired of congratulating all my friends on their babies while my arms remained empty, tired of carrying the incredible guilt of not giving my husband the child he so desperately wanted. I wanted to beat the odds and hold my baby. I wanted to leave behind my life as an infertility victim and become an infertility survivor.

Having embarked on this painful journey, I knew others must feel as lost, tired and as alone as we did. Once a very private and reserved person, I gathered my strength and openly shared our journey on the Internet. Word after word was typed as needle after needle pierced my skin; paragraph after paragraph took shape as ultrasound after ultrasound monitored our progress. It was an amazing milestone to finally post on our Web site that we were indeed pregnant.

Achieving success with our first IVF cycle changed our lives forever. We have been given the chance to experience one of life's greatest joys, raising our son. Along the path to parenthood, we have met some of the most wonderful and courageous people: fellow IVFers and fellow infertility survivors. None of us knew our destiny when we began our journey, but we all shared that desire deep within our souls to carry us to the end.

Becoming a mother has ignited my desire to write this book in hopes of bringing to light the very emotional aspect of infertility and the treatments which allow us to hold our dreams tightly to our hearts. I write this book not as a physician but rather as a woman who realizes so many others face the same demons I once did. I write this book to reach those still desperately needing a sign that they are not alone and to encourage them as they work to overcome the obstacles set before them. I write this book as a testament that medical science applied with a caring hand can bring incredible beauty into this world that will span many generations.

Often the voices of the infertile population are lost in the roar of the "naturally" conceiving population. Within these pages lies a message of beauty and love, of hope and inspiration, all possible because of in vitro fertilization. This isn't how I planned my life. This isn't the path I would have chosen. But it is a journey that has forever changed me and I truly hope by sharing my struggle, those still chasing their dreams will find the strength they need to see them through the dark days of trying to conceive.

Three simple letters: IVF. No simple task to undertake, but truly an amazing opportunity to create life where once all seemed lost and to finally feel blessed after suffering through heartache and disappointment.

PART ONE

Our Journey to Parenthood

Chapter One

Struggling with Infertility

To meet your best friend and love of your life at the tender age of thirteen seems inconceivable, yet it marks the beginning of my story. Jeff and I both felt early in our relationship that we had found our soul mate. We graduated high school together, got engaged and soon faced our first challenge as a couple: Separation. Jeff enlisted in the United States Navy and left for the East Coast while I packed up and left for college. It was in a blustery ice storm my sophomore year of college that we vowed to cherish and love one another for a lifetime. Although the miles between us made newlywed life difficult, Jeff continued to live on the East Coast as he finished his three-year stint while I continued my college studies here in the Midwest. My fourth year of college found us finally living together, preparing to move to the suburbs of Chicago where I would attend medical school. It was during my first year of medical school that I went off my birth control pills. Jeff and I entertained the thought of starting our family, but after trying for one month, decided it would be best to wait a few more years. After all, we were still young and had plenty of time.

Four years later, during the fifth month of my family practice residency we began actively trying for a baby again. By now we had bought our first home and felt ready to take on the tremendous responsibility of raising a child. At the same time, a heavy call schedule and dissatisfaction with my residency program were starting to wear on me. The doubts I had during medical school about clinical medicine being the right career choice were troubling my mind more and more. To help another human being in a time of need was a feeling unlike no other, but I was being asked to sacrifice so much of myself in order to do this. In the seventh month of my family practice residency, near the end of a grueling obstetrics rotation, I took a leave of absence from the program in order to clear my head and decide once and for all if clinical medicine really was right for me.

Six weeks later I found myself standing in the bathroom with a home pregnancy test in hand. I had been feeling different and was spotting mid-cycle. Without my heavy call schedule our baby making efforts had been unhindered, so pregnancy was definitely a possibility. Even so, I was amazed to see the positive test sitting on the counter when I returned. I remember jumping up and down yelling, "We're pregnant, we're pregnant" much to the amusement of our dog. Wanting to surprise Jeff, I ran out to the store, bought a pacifier and disguised it as an early Valentine's Day gift. Poor Jeff barely got through the door before I was shoving the bag into his hands.

"No way," spilled from Jeff's mouth as he removed the pacifier. We both reached to touch my belly and smiled. We had always envisioned ourselves surrounded by the pitter-patter of little feet and now it seemed our dreams were coming true. We spent most the night celebrating the wonderful news, talking of things to come, holding each other close. Little did we know how quickly our dream would fade.

Over the next three days my spotting and cramping worsened. The inner voice that first spoke only of exciting things to come began to whisper of doubts and uncertainty. My tears of joy were replaced with tears of sadness as the threat of miscarriage weighed heavily on my mind. Our first trip to the obstetrician was less than comforting. My hCG level was low for how far along I was in the pregnancy and I was told I was likely losing the baby. A couple days later my hCG level rose, but too slowly for a normal pregnancy and the obstetrician was unable to locate the baby on ultrasound. My spotting increased with bright red blood at times and I began to have sharp pains rather than cramping. Three days later, when another blood test showed my hCG level to still be rising but still too slowly, I was scheduled for a vaginal ultrasound at the hospital.

Through it all, Jeff and I tried to stay positive that things would work out, but on the day of the ultrasound my pain was sharper and my bleeding was more pronounced. When the radiologist entered the room to discuss our ultrasound results, our hearts sank as he spoke the words "ectopic pregnancy." The baby had a heartbeat but had implanted in my right Fallopian tube, which was now close to bursting. I wasn't allowed to leave the hospital. I stood sobbing in the hospital lobby as I phoned my sister to tell her we were pregnant but that I was being admitted for emergency surgery to remove the baby from my tube. I couldn't stop the tears even as they wheeled me into the operating room, moved me onto the table, and placed the mask over my face. February 1, 1996 was a turning point in our lives for more than one reason. It was the day we lost our first baby at seven weeks gestation, heart still beating. It was the day we found a deeper love for each other through heartache. And, although we did not know it at the time, it was the day we lost the ability to conceive unassisted.

Jeff Remembers

After I learned the hCG levels weren't rising the way they should, I could immediately feel my heart being squeezed by sorrow. I honestly didn't realize what the pregnancy meant to me until it was being taken away from me. During the ultrasound I prayed that the numbers were wrong, but they weren't. My prayer went unanswered. Why? Why us? The only thing I could do was to console Jen. I was helpless.

In the morning I had been a mother-to-be, hoping for the best. By the evening I was an ICU patient grieving for my child. My laparoscopic surgery had been converted to an open abdominal surgery, leaving me with a large incision, excessive blood loss, and unbelievable pain. Jeff spent the night by my side, comforting me when I would briefly awaken, assuring me everything would be okay, and gently wiping the tears as they rolled down my face. The next day I was stable enough to be moved out of the ICU. My body was already beginning to heal but my heart and soul would not be so quick to follow. I cried for the incredible emptiness inside me, I cried for the terrible pain throughout my body. I cried for the injustice of it all.

The day after my surgery Jeff ran into our neighbor in the hospital, there with his wife who had just delivered their third child. The second day after my surgery, the condolence calls and flowers from friends and family started to arrive. By the third day I was lost in my grief, wanting only to be home and away from everyone.

My recovery was painful but fairly quick. Within a week I was scrubbing floors, cleaning windows, doing anything to keep my mind occupied. Nights were the worst. I needed help in and out of bed and sleep was usually slow to come, leaving plenty of time to think. In the wee hours of one insomnia-ridden night, I decided to leave my residency. Most wouldn't understand that decision, but I just couldn't go back to a place where the call schedule and placement of my desk were more important than the terrible loss I was dealing with.

The next year was difficult to say the least. I found myself consuming food as a way to deal with my pain. Although we were instructed to wait a few months before trying to conceive again, Jeff and I started immediately following my first period. I still remember our first few baby-making efforts being painful with my scar still so new. We had been told following surgery that, although they had saved my right tube, it would likely become blocked with adhesions (fibrous tissue resulting from an inflammatory response). My left tube, we were told, appeared completely normal, so we should be able to become pregnant again. Had our surgeon been honest at the time and told us how my surgery had been botched, leaving my left tube damaged, we might have been spared painful testing. But he didn't and we walked out feeling hope that we could become pregnant again if given enough time.

I became consumed by the need to become pregnant in order to heal the incredible pain in my heart. One month passed, then another, then another. Each month I found myself pacing in the bathroom while I waited for the home pregnancy test to turn positive, sinking to the floor in tears when it came up negative time after time. Of course, in hindsight, I realize stress was making my period start late. But at the time I saw every late day and every turn of my stomach as a glimmer of hope. Month after month, I swore not to buy that dreaded pee test, and month after month, our wastebasket stood as a testament to my failure. More times than I would like to admit, not one but two, and sometimes three, home pregnancy tests sat glaring at me, all negative.

I soon fell into the vicious cycle most women battling infertility fall into: dedicating all my energy to achieving pregnancy, feeling confident that this month was going to be the month, placing all my hope in a piece of plastic, and tumbling down into a pit of anger and self-pity when my period arrived, only to start all over again the following month. After several months of trying to conceive, we scheduled an appointment with our gynecologist again. Frustrated by our lack of success and my continued pelvic pain so many months after surgery, Jeff and I hoped our doctor could give us the answers we desperately needed. His concern at the time was that excessive adhesions were contributing to both my pain and inability to conceive, possibly blocking my Fallopian tube. I underwent exploratory laparoscopic surgery and my doctor removed dense adhesions encircling my right tube. After surgery, he encouraged us to continue our baby-making efforts.

Four weeks later, we found ourselves back at the hospital, this time for a hysterosalpingogram (HSG), a dye test that reveals if the Fallopian tubes are open or blocked. A normal HSG will demonstrate dye spilling from both Fallopian tubes. My HSG showed my right tube to be blocked at the halfway point and my left tube to be blocked at the point where it attaches to the uterus. News that my right tube was blocked was not surprising. Adhesions commonly reform following surgery. We were not prepared to hear the disheartening news that my left tube was also blocked, especially after being told it appeared normal following both my surgeries. If only our doctor had been honest with us, we would have been prepared.

We returned home in very low spirits. I crawled into bed to relax and think about the results and our next possible option while Jeff went out to mow the lawn. By time he came back to check on me thirty minutes later, I was in excruciating pain. It felt as if a knife was twisting and slicing through me. The pain was intense and overpowering, similar to the pain after surgery for my ectopic pregnancy. Nothing I did seemed to help. Jeff frantically phoned our doctor, fearing something was terribly wrong. He was informed that some women experience significant pain following an HSG, especially when the tubes are both blocked. The nurse assured him the pain would slowly pass and instructed us to use pain medication as needed. I lay in bed, rocking gently back and forth with my head resting on Jeff's lap, crying until I had no tears left to cry. Three hours later, the pain had dulled and I found peace in sleep until morning.

Since my right tube had closed within four weeks following surgery, it was unlikely it would remain open for any length of time, even with further surgery. It seemed my right tube was a lost cause. However, our physician wanted to attempt tuboplasty of my left tube, a fairly new procedure at the time used for tubal blockage occurring so close to the uterus. The procedure involved placing a catheter through my cervix, snaking it into the left tube, and inflating a balloon in order to open the tube, much as they do with angioplasty of the heart.

Jeff and I agreed to try the tuboplasty procedure in the hopes we would be able to conceive on our own.

Once again, I found myself back at the hospital, lying on a cold table in radiology, hoping for a positive outcome. The pain of the tuboplasty procedure was unbearable. I had been instructed to take two ibuprofen tablets prior to arriving at the hospital, so I had expected only some minor cramping. I dug my nails into my palms to the point of bleeding and ground my teeth to keep from screaming. Sweat poured from me and I soon felt nauseous and lightheaded. After fifteen minutes I couldn't stand the pain any longer and asked my doctor to stop. He asked me to hang in there; he was still trying to maneuver the catheter into the tube and didn't want to give up just yet. I begged him to stop and started crying, "Please stop. Please stop. I can't stand it." Finally he abandoned the procedure and allowed me to sit up. I immediately began heaving from the pain and slumped into Jeff's arms.

Back at home and back into bed, where I lay sobbing with pain from the procedure, riddled with guilt for asking our doctor to stop. If I could have held out just a little longer and tolerated the pain a few more minutes, we might be able to conceive unassisted. Instead, we were scheduled for a consultation with a reproductive endocrinologist to discuss further surgical options and in vitro fertilization.

Jeff Remembers

I was sitting outside radiology when the tuboplasty started. Within minutes I could hear Jen crying and begging the doctor to stop. I jumped from my chair and was at the door in one step. I heard Jen again telling the doctor to stop, but I didn't go in. Both hands on the door with my head hung low and tears in my eyes, my mind started to wonder. Is her pain right now worth having a child? Could the doctor do what he said he could do? Isn't there anyway this could be done without pain? Then I was snapped back into reality with Jen's third scream. I immediately went in and yelled at the doctor to stop. It was over. I held Jen in my arms, wiping her tears. Again, I was helpless to do anything else.

By now the pain and stress of battling our infertility were taking their toll. No matter how hard I tried to focus on the other aspects of my life, achieving pregnancy seemed to take center stage. I had a medical degree and knew both of my Fallopian tubes were blocked, yet each month I prayed that my period would not arrive. I rationalized that there was always the chance my tubes would spontaneously open. Miracles happen all the time, right? Our friends and neighbors continued to add to their families as Jeff and I stood with empty arms. It all seemed so unfair.

Our consultation with the reproductive endocrinologist was not encouraging. With my history of an ectopic pregnancy, we were not good candidates for stent placement in either tube (a procedure to help hold the tube open) and our insurance at the time was a self-funded policy. This meant the carrier could refuse coverage for any fertility treatments, such as in vitro fertilization—which they did. I had the debt of a physician without the income of a physician, so it was financially impossible for us to pay out of pocket for in vitro.

Library Resource Center
Renton Technical College
3000 N.E. 4th St.
Renton, WA 98056

We found ourselves facing another turning point in our lives. We could either continue struggling with our infertility or we could walk away for awhile and allow our battle wounds to heal. I was tired of crying every month when my period started. I was tired of answering the dreaded question of "When are you going to have kids?" I was tired of judging all the good and bad in my life by my ability or inability to get pregnant. Buying a home pregnancy test, knowing full well I had blocked tubes, was insane. Hiding them from Jeff to avoid talking about my obsession was unhealthy. I couldn't live my life like that anymore. I took a long look in the mirror one day and didn't like the person staring back at me. I was extremely overweight, I was full of self-pity, and I was angry at the world for every unwanted pregnancy, every fertile Myrtle, every flippant remark from fertile friends about God choosing those who should and shouldn't have children.

I sat down with Jeff and we had a very emotional heart-to-heart. We both had to be okay with the decision to not have children, whether it was for a few years or for a lifetime. The decision was difficult to make, but we agreed to put our relationship back on center stage in our lives. We both set our minds to losing weight, enjoying life as a couple, and spending time with friends. No more home pregnancy tests and no more beating ourselves up over something we couldn't control. But I had to do more than just say the words, I had to live them. Every infertile woman has vowed to live at least one month free of the baby-making obsession, but few of us are able to hold true to ourselves. I knew that realistically I would never be able to live two to three years without thinking about a child or what we had already endured. But I felt strongly that I needed to push all these things to the back of my mind and not allow them to cloud my life every day. Not an easy task, but it was best for Jeff and best for me.

A year passed and life was good. We both dropped the extra pounds weighing us down. We socialized with friends. We did so many of the things we always talked about doing. I found enjoyment doing activities with my friends, their children and my nephew. Did I ever have bad days? Most definitely. News of someone becoming pregnant was always difficult. I would be filled with happiness for them but memories of our loss and struggle would always come rushing to the surface. But rather than drowning in them as before, I allowed them to wash over me.

Six more months down the line, my heart again began to whisper, "I long for a child." I had met an obstetrician/gynecologist, who also had a medical management company, and I began working for him out of his OB/GYN office. Some days were almost unbearable as I stood watching all the pregnant bellies go by, wanting to waddle down the hall as they all did. I was more in love with Jeff than ever and we were having so much fun together, but something was missing. I knew deep down that there was a strong possibility we might never hear that pitter-patter of little feet, but I needed to at least try.

My body and mind felt so much stronger than before and I felt confident I was ready to endure more testing, more surgery, and more pain, if necessary. Jeff wasn't quite as ready as I was, though. He still wanted a child, but hoped to wait another year or two. At the time I was a little resentful but now I realize our journey up to that point had been hard on him as well. I felt we needed to start planning for the future, though, so Jeff left a job filled with wonderful friends to start somewhere new with insurance covering in vitro.

Chapter Two

Cycling to Realize Our Dream

In June of 2000, yet another turning point in our lives arrived. As we drove home from a baseball game with our nephew who was visiting for the weekend, Jeff had tears in his eyes. Watching all of the fathers with their sons and daughters had really affected him. Jeff seemed so certain that he would never have the opportunity to share a baseball game with his own child. After tucking our nephew in for the night, we sat and talked about what the future held for us. Although we knew it would be a difficult path to take, we both felt this empty space in our lives and felt ready to attempt in vitro fertilization.

Jeff Remembers

At the time I was very happy with our lives. We were very social with our friends and family. I don't even remember the last time I had thought of having a child. But one baseball game changed all of that. I witnessed dozens of boys and girls sharing popcorn and cotton candy with their mothers and fathers. It hit me like a truck; I wanted to be a dad! I wanted to

teach my son how to throw a curve ball. I wanted to
show my daughter how to play hopscotch. All the
feelings I had years ago came flooding back to me
within nine innings of a baseball game. Anger set in
on the way home from the game. Why can't we have
a child?! Anger, not at Jen, but at God. What could I
have possibly done in my life to not deserve a child?

———————

The next morning, I dug out the insurance packet and began
reading through our plan coverage. Much to my dismay, I found
in bold type that in vitro fertilization was not covered. Okay,
this was a bump in the road but nothing that required a detour.
I discussed our situation with a colleague who called a
reproductive endocrinologist he went to school with. My hope
was that we might be able to work out some sort of payment
plan. The consultation did not go well, though. I felt like the
five hundredth patient on a long list of other patients. Great
emphasis was placed on paying up front for everything; no
special payment plans were offered. I left the consultation
feeling like we had just been run off the road to parenthood.

Four weeks later, I mentioned to my boss how discouraging
my consultation had been and he told me of a reproductive
endocrinologist they referred many of their patients to.
Although I knew we didn't have the funds, that inner voice
pushed me. Two weeks later, Jeff and I walked into the office of
a reproductive endocrinologist (RE) for a consultation. His
office had taken the time to contact our insurance company
directly and found everything was covered with co-pays except
the actual in vitro fertilization procedure itself and the
cryopreservation procedure, if needed. That meant all the

medications and monitoring would be covered. That news put a permanent smile on my face for days.

I immediately liked our RE. He walked in with a smile and a handshake. He spent a lot of time explaining in vitro fertilization and what lay ahead for us. With our medical history, he gave us about a 50 percent chance of getting pregnant with our first cycle. My heart raced when we learned the entire process would take approximately six weeks from start to finish. "Wow," I thought. "We're really going to do this." We walked out in high spirits, holding hands, loaded down with paperwork and consent forms.

We arrived home and I immediately read every page, trying to absorb the entire process. With so many opportunities for things to go wrong, for side effects, and for failure, I must admit I was a little scared. But our reproductive endocrinologist had spoken with such confidence and resolve and we were ideal candidates for in vitro fertilization. At that time I was blissfully ignorant of all the couples in our exact circumstances who were still cycling after being labeled ideal candidates and having perfect cycles. We read every consent form that night and went to bed feeling lighter in our hearts than we had in many years.

Jen's Journal Entry 09-19-2000

This is the closest we've been to realizing our dream of a little one. The possible risk of cancer with the medications scares me the most. I immediately liked our RE. He has a wonderful attitude/bedside manner and comes very highly recommended. I feel comfortable enough with him to discuss anything and everything regarding our upcoming cycle.

Jeff's Online Blog Entry

I have a pretty easy road compared to Jen. I had no idea there were so many potential problems and side effects from the medications and procedures. Not to mention the chance that they might use the wrong sperm or implant the wrong embryos. I guess the biggest preparation for me is to really look myself in the face and say, yes, I am ready to do this. It means we will both have to make sacrifices. I'll be putting in some overtime and helping more at home. I know I need to be ready to help out wherever I can because from what I've read, some of the medications are going to be rough on Jen.

The next day I began searching the World Wide Web for informative sites on the process of in vitro. I browsed through clinic site after clinic site. They all explained the procedure in great detail and provided wonderful photos of developing follicles, eggs, sperm and embryos, but most were so technical and detailed, even I had a difficult time understanding everything. The success rates were very discouraging and it seemed no site really hit upon what it really felt like to go through a cycle. That night, as I sat talking with Jeff about all of the sites and information, I decided to take on the task of creating a Web site that would outline the process in general and would share all the emotions during our cycle. I was surprised by how quickly the name came to me: Hope with IVF. Three words which speak volumes to those struggling to conceive. Building the site from scratch would educate me on what lay ahead for us and would occupy my mind during the long weeks ahead, or at least I hoped.

We decided early on we would not tell our families about our cycle. We knew if our cycle went smoothly, we would be testing before Christmas and we couldn't think of a nicer surprise than telling everyone we were pregnant. We did tell some of our closer friends since we knew our social life would be slowing down dramatically during our cycle. My boss and co-workers already knew about our cycle and Jeff decided to tell his boss and the facility director. We vowed to each other that we were going down this path together, so Jeff planned to give me every single injection and planned to be present at as many of my ultrasounds as possible.

Since Jeff had never had a semen analysis done, we were scheduled for that test first. We arrived at the office together and sat waiting for the room to become available. I joked with Jeff the entire time, asking if he wanted any help or if he could handle this one. He kept a very good sense of humor about the entire thing and assured me he was capable of taking this test all on his own. We waited for quite awhile, apparently the couple before us was having a difficult time in there. Finally, Jeff was taken back to the collection room while I sat reading a magazine. It seemed a long time before Jeff returned, but in actuality it was probably only about fifteen to twenty minutes. I asked if everything had gone all right. Jeff smiled, telling me not to worry—he had done his duty.

On the ride home, we joked about the whole thing. Apparently, they had pretty good "study aids" in the room, but Jeff got a little side-tracked for a few minutes. Leave it to my husband to pick up a Victoria's Secret catalog to look for clothes and lingerie for me. He said he flipped through the entire thing, picking out outfits he thought I would like, before he realized he was a little off track. After all, he was there for a specific reason. He put the catalog down and got back to business. It is definitely one of the more humorous memories of our cycle. Jeff's semen analysis came back normal and our hepatitis and HIV tests came back negative. So far, so good.

Jeff Remembers

There is only one word for this experience:
UNCOMFORTABLE!

Since we already knew that both of my Fallopian tubes were blocked, I thankfully did not need to have another HSG. I did have a hysterosonogram to check the anatomy of my uterus. The hysterosonogram was pretty uncomfortable, but tolerable. The procedure is fairly simple. Fluid is injected inside the uterus through the cervix and then an ultrasound is performed to look at the uterine lining and structure. I had some moderate cramping when the fluid was injected, more painful than menstrual cramping, but nothing as bad as my HSG. Unfortunately, our RE noticed a questionable area on the ultrasound. It was difficult to determine if the spot was simply the normal anatomy of my uterus, or if it was a growth, as in a fibroid or polyp. It looked like a fibroid in one view but then appeared to be part of the wall of my uterus in two other views. Our doctor felt it would be better to delay the start of our cycle in order to do a hysteroscopy, which would allow him to visualize the inside of my uterus directly.

This same question had been raised by the radiologist who had read my HSG films a couple years back. At that time he had concluded the area was part of my normal uterine anatomy. I mentioned this to our RE. He instructed me to bring in the films so that he could review them himself and told me that we should decide if we wanted to proceed as planned or delay our cycle in order to do the hysteroscopy. Jeff and I walked out of the office somewhat dejected, facing yet another difficult decision.

I have always been a strong believer when it comes to listening to your inner voice or woman's intuition—whatever name you'd like to give it. My intuition had never steered me wrong in the past. When we left the office, my inner voice was nearly shouting, "Do not postpone your cycle!" I had such a strong feeling that this cycle would work and that we needed to stay on course. I talked things over with Jeff and expressed my feelings to him. Jeff left the decision to me and said he would support whatever choice I made. I dropped off my HSG films three days later and asked the nurse to relay to our doctor that we wanted to continue with our cycle as originally planned.

On October 20, 2000, we began our first in vitro fertilization cycle. The intense emotions on that first night of injections are difficult to describe. I felt excited, scared, happy, terrified. There is nothing quite like wanting something so intensely that when opportunity arrives, you're almost sick to your stomach.

Jen's Online Blog Entry

We started Lupron injections on 10/20/00. My progesterone level that morning showed I had ovulated and our RE gave us the green light. That night was so exciting yet so scary. Jeff and I decided to split responsibility for the Lupron injections. I drew up the medication and chose the site of injection, and he actually gave me the injection.

In the morning, I took my first baby aspirin (I took a baby aspirin each day of our cycle) and counted the hours until our first injection. The Lupron injection signaled the official start of our cycle and would suppress my ovaries and prevent ovulation. Despite all our nervousness and anxiety, my first Lupron injection went smoothly. I drew up the medication and prepared the injection spot, and Jeff did the actual injection into my stomach. Jeff's hands were shaking just a bit, but he did a wonderful job. The whole experience was almost anticlimactic. The injection was completely painless. I had some itching for several minutes, and then nothing. No cheering, no fireworks, no balloons dropping from the ceiling; just Jeff, the dog, and me, back to watching television. Oh, how quickly things would change!

Jeff Remembers

Needles have never bothered me for some reason, so giving Jen her shots made me feel like I was contributing to this cycle. I was nervous on the first one, but I must have done okay because she didn't hit or kick me.

By the fifth Lupron injection, my life started to turn. It wasn't anything I could put my finger on, but somehow I felt a little off.

I found myself crying at commercials, feeling depressed, overwhelmed, and sometimes feeling downright angry at the world for no apparent reason. Poor Jeff never knew what woman would greet him at the door. The Lupron injections were actually hurting by now. An injection placed too far to the side, too high or too low would sting a lot, so Jeff only had a limited area to work with. Even with alternating the injection site, my stomach was sore. I began dreading our nightly injection ritual.

Jeff's Online Blog Entry

Poor Jen has had a rough time with the Lupron. Her headaches have been pretty rough on her. My last few injections have hurt her and we have plenty more to go. I'm hanging in there as best I can on this wild roller-coaster ride. I keep reminding myself she's at the mercy of her hormones and how close we are to a baby. She's been craving affection, so I'm giving Jen extra hugs and they have put a smile back on her face.

Our days were still pretty normal, however. I worked on our Web site and continued with my regular work schedule. Jeff continued with his work schedule as well. I found myself staying in more and more as we continued the Lupron injections (again, meant to suppress my ovaries and prevent ovulation). I vividly remember running out to the store for some odds and ends. No big deal, I planned to pick up just a few things and be on my way. I walked aisle after aisle, popping things into my cart and marking off my list. Halfway down my list was laundry detergent. Okay, that was just right around the corner. I found myself standing in the laundry detergent aisle searching and searching. Every detergent known to man sat on the shelf, but my particular brand was nowhere to be seen. I moved boxes and bottles to check the back of the shelf, stood on tiptoe to see what was up on the very top shelf. Nothing. In that instant, I completely lost it. I think I called the store every swear word I knew, not once, but twice and out loud, for God and everyone to hear. The world was weighing on my shoulders already and now, to top it off, I couldn't even complete a simple task like buying laundry detergent.

After about five minutes of intense anger and swearing, I stopped myself cold. I was stunned by my reaction to say the least. What was wrong with me? I kept waiting to hear over the intercom, "Security to the laundry detergent aisle immediately. We have a madwoman on the loose!" Thankfully, no one had witnessed or heard my embarrassing tirade. I took a deep breath, walked out of the aisle, went straight to check out and then home. When Jeff arrived home that night I proclaimed myself banned from solo shopping until the Lupron injections were finished. After hearing what happened, Jeff agreed it was an excellent idea.

As I write this now I am smiling about my shopping misadventure, but it was anything but funny that day. It was so unlike me to overact, and it kind of scared me to have such hate and anger inside all over some lousy laundry detergent. Obviously the Lupron was doing its job. My estrogen levels were dropping and I was getting my first taste of the wild fluctuations of menopause.

Soon the insomnia set in. Some nights I lay awake in bed for hours, waiting for sleep to come. Most nights I was haunted by nightmares of screwing up our cycle. I would dream of forgetting to do an injection or incorrectly mixing the medication. The injections, the insomnia, the nightmares, the bickering over unimportant matters: These things made nighttime the worst part of our cycle. Although, I must admit, some nights it was as if we were back to ourselves, laughing, joking and talking about everyday things. Regardless of what our day or night was like, when bedtime arrived, we would lie in bed snuggling. The moments of tenderness between us during the suppression phase were what kept me going.

I also found myself bombarded with terrible headaches. Unlike the other side effects, the headaches seemed worse during the day. No amount of Tylenol or Advil could ease those headaches. The only thing that helped me was sleep. Luckily, my flexible work schedule allowed me to catch a nap here and there on really bad days. If I felt the world weighed on my shoulders before, it was crushing me now. I stopped talking about having a baby. It seemed as if the obstacles before us were insurmountable. My enthusiasm about a positive cycle was quickly fading. All I seemed to think about was getting through the next injection. I felt as if I had been on Lupron for months rather than twelve days and with no end in sight.

Yet one glorious day—November 1, to be exact—I awoke to my period. For the first time since trying to conceive, I was thrilled to see red. What had once stood as glaring proof of failure now signaled a positive turn. I called the office and they asked me to come in immediately for an ultrasound. My sister was due to arrive in two hours on her way in to have lunch with me to celebrate her birthday a day early, so I had to scramble. My ultrasound showed my ovaries to be free of cysts. I had blood work drawn to check my estrogen and luteinizing hormone (LH) levels which would indicate if my ovaries were suppressed enough to start the next phase of our cycle. I rushed back home, just beating my sister. I made up some excuse about falling asleep on the bed to explain why I wasn't ready, smiling inside at my little secret. I had a nice day with my sister and then returned home to wait for my lab results. Later that night, the call came. My estrogen (E2) level came back at 68 and my luteinizing hormone (LH) level came back at 4, showing that my ovaries were indeed suppressed. I was overjoyed to hear the words, "No more Lupron."

Jen's Online Blog Entry

We've finished our Lupron and all I have to say is, "Thank God!" Incredible mood swings, nasty headaches, nightly insomnia, and look at me wrong and I'm crying. The last few shots started to hurt so we're going to move on to the thighs and deltoids (upper arm) with the stimulation phase. IVF is definitely not an easy road but we are a third of the way there. My labs came back showing I am suppressed and my ultrasound showed my ovaries to be cyst-free...so 11/01/00 is my first Gonal-F injection.

On the evening of November 1, 2000, Jeff gave me my first injection of Gonal-F, 4 amps subcutaneously (beneath the skin) and the stimulation phase officially began. We decided to inject my upper arm in order to give my poor stomach a much needed break from needles. I was feeling more and more like a pincushion and my stomach was sore, even during the day. The Gonal-F injections were more difficult than the Lupron injections. There was quite a bit more medication to be injected and they stung more than the Lupron. After my fourth injection of Gonal-F, I returned to the office for another ultrasound and more blood work. The ultrasound showed that my ovaries weren't doing much as far as developing follicles and my blood work showed my E2 level was 73. We were instructed to continue with the 4 amps of Gonal-F a night. Because the stomach is so vascular, Jeff and I decided to go back to injecting my stomach in hopes of getting my E2 level to rise more quickly.

Jen's Online Blog Entry

I am so grateful we are able to attempt this, but IVF is very draining on both your mind and body. My ovaries have lots of follicles but they have plenty of growing left to do. I get a lot of stabbing pains from both ovaries and everything seems so overwhelming now with my hormones the way they are. And, of course, fewer of my clothes fit the further we get through our cycle. I'm having at least two to three nightmares about forgetting something or doing something wrong with my IVF each night that startle me awake. I can't wait to have a peaceful night's sleep again. I still spend several hours a day thinking about a baby and hoping this will bring us a sweet angel all our own. Next week we should be ready for our egg retrieval and that will be here before we know it.

Jeff's Online Blog Entry

Stress, stress, and more stress. Most of the time I'm not really sure what to do or say to make Jen feel better. I'm trying to be as supportive as I can, but, at this point, I think I would cry too if I saw another needle coming at me. You'd like to hurry so the injection is finished quicker, but that just hurts more, so I just keep my hand steady and try not to jiggle the needle if Jen is crying. Considering how easy I have it compared to Jen, I am surprised at how emotionally drained I feel. It's really tough being the one to inflict pain on someone you love so much. It really kind of tears you apart inside to want a baby so bad but to have to watch your wife suffer to get there without any guarantee of success.

At first I thought Jen had lost her desire to go through with this; she doesn't talk about a baby much lately. But now I realize she is focusing on getting through the next day of pain and the next injection. Don't get me wrong, it's not all bad. We're still laughing and joking together, but when 9 o'clock rolls around I see a change come over her, almost like that long sigh gives her the strength to get up and grab the medication from the cupboard. But all in all, we're hanging in there!

At this point, I had been on Gonal-F for five nights and my headaches were already improving. I was able to fall asleep at night and my nightmares of messing up my cycle were replaced with dreams of a baby. I had a recurring dream of myself gazing upon a tightly wrapped bundle, smiling as sunlight streamed in through the window. Although the Lupron side effects were vanishing, it became more difficult to prepare myself for the nightly injection ritual. My stomach felt extremely tender and, no matter how gentle Jeff tried to be, each injection hurt more and more. I often cried as the needle punctured my skin while I tried hard to hold still and get through the injection as best as possible. The stress of our cycle was starting to affect me. I didn't feel like socializing at all and each day I felt like I had been put through the wringer the night before. Even my mother was asking if I was okay. I held fast to our promise, though, and said I was fighting a virus.

After seven nights of Gonal-F injections, I went in for more monitoring. My ovaries were producing follicles of a good size now, ranging from 8 to 11 mm. My blood work showed my E2 level had jumped to 243 and my endometrial lining was up to 10.2 mm. Our goal was to thicken my lining to at least 11 mm and to get as many of my follicles to a size of 15-18 mm. It seemed we were headed in the right direction. Finally, some progress!

My arms were so bruised from all the blood draws, I stopped wearing short sleeves. On the night of our eighth Gonal-F injection, I told Jeff that I couldn't take another needle. He hugged me and told me what a great job I was doing and how close we were to a baby. And really, what choice did I have? I realized there was no way I was going to stop now, so I laid down on the couch, exposed my stomach and sobbed as more Gonal-F went into my body.

During the day my spirits were better, especially compared to the days of Lupron. I was released from my solo shopping ban and tried to get back into the swing of things. I felt some twinges of pain and some soreness from my ovaries—all to be expected with several follicles growing inside. Two more nights of Gonal-F and I was back in the office for more blood work. I felt as if my entire life revolved around needles. They were either stealing from me or injecting me. I began to develop a strong hatred of them. Yellow, black and blue, with a sore stomach, I sat at home waiting for my test results. My E2 level came back at 479 and my LH was at 1. We wanted my LH level as low as possible to prevent ovulation and needed my estrogen level to keep rising, so we were right on track. My ultrasound that morning showed my endometrial lining was 11.4 mm and my follicles were increasing both in size and number. Okay. I hurt. I was emotionally drained. I wasn't fitting into my clothes as well anymore. But, I could finally see light at the end of the tunnel.

I felt like "The Little Engine that Could": "I think I can, I think I can, I think I can...make it through this cycle." The twinges from my ovaries were now stabbing pains that stole my breath away at times. I willingly stayed home more because walking too much brought the pain on. I was happy and ready to take on the world again, but my body did not feel so well anymore. What kind of cruel joke is this, I thought. When my body was willing and able my mind was a wreck, and once my mind caught up, my body was on the downslide. One positive note was that the Gonal-F injections didn't bother me as much anymore. Funny how knowing you only face a few more injection nights can make everything more tolerable. I began the Gonal-F countdown. I estimated we would likely have four more nights of Gonal-F and then the stimulation phase would be over.

The morning following my eleventh night of Gonal-F found me once again at the office for another ultrasound and more blood work. Come on follies, I thought. Grow, grow, grow!

Much to my surprise, that is exactly what my follicles had been doing in the last couple of days. They filled the ultrasound screen and ranged from 15 mm to 18 mm. My endometrial lining was 12.3 mm. Wow! We did it! No wonder I hurt so much. My ovaries were filled with lots of large follicles just waiting for the next phase in our cycle. Our RE spoke those glorious words: No more Gonal-F injections. We were instructed to complete three tasks that night: hCG trigger shot to be given at 7:00 P.M., take my first dose of Doxycycline at night, and sexual intercourse.

Jen's Journal Entry 11-12-2000

We are two-thirds of the way there! My mood has been better the last few days and coming to the end of the stimulation phase just makes everything rosy! Please God, let this work for us…we're so ready to be a mommy and daddy!

The timing and administration of the hCG trigger shot was important. Our retrieval was timed to occur thirty-six hours after the hCG trigger. We needed to make sure that all of the medication was injected into the muscle at 7:00 P.M. The four tablets of Doxycycline were spread out over thirty-six hours and were important to protect against infection from the invasive retrieval procedure. Having sexual intercourse with ejaculation was key to ensuring a fresh sample from Jeff on retrieval day. More importantly, I think it was crucial to maintaining our sanity. The process so far had been clinical—lots of numbers, lots of needles and lots of monitoring. With me suffering from so many medication side effects, there hadn't been much room for romance.

That evening we spent the night as lovers rather than IVFers. My E2 level was 1449 and my LH was 3. We said goodbye to the stimulation phase and moved towards the retrieval stage, and it was such a relief to both of us. We had thirty-six hours to enjoy without the stress of mixing medications, injecting my stomach or counting numbers. They were an incredible thirty-six hours indeed.

Our retrieval was scheduled for November 14, 2000, at 6:30 A.M. I had a difficult time sleeping the night before. I felt very apprehensive about the procedure. I worried it would be very painful. I mean, the thought of a large needle inserted into my ovaries several times to withdraw eggs was not a pleasant one. I finally drifted off to sleep only to wake up twice from nightmares of not making it to our appointment. At 3:30 A.M., November 14, I was awake and getting ready. We left early in case we ran into any problems getting to the clinic. We arrived at 5:45 A.M. and sat in the waiting area with another couple. We smiled at them, they smiled back. Each of us tried to be supportive but knew full well we were all a little anxious. Jeff was very cool, calm and collected. I was extremely nervous. I kept wringing my hands and pacing the room to calm down. The nurses finally called me back to the prep room just after six o'clock.

I thought Jeff would be in the room with me, but he was instructed to wait up front. Once they had me prepped, he would be called back to their collection room in order to provide his semen sample to be used for fertilization. I went from nervous to scared to death in a matter of minutes. As I got into the gown and onto the table, memories of my ectopic surgery came rushing back. I needed Jeff in the room so badly for support, but he had his own part to play out that day.

Just when I began feeling overwhelmed by the situation, our doctor walked in with a smile. He touched my arm and spoke with me about his recent trip to Florida where he spoke at a conference. The conversation was exactly what I needed at the time. He asked if I was feeling the medication they had put into my IV and I said, "No." Two minutes later, my head started to cloud a little. I remember saying that I could feel the medication now and the next thing I knew, I was opening my eyes to Jeff sitting by my side. I immediately smiled and reached for him. Jeff asked how I felt and told me the procedure was over.

I felt very sore and tried to sit up. My head immediately began spinning and I felt a wave of nausea sweep over me. I lay back down for a few more minutes and tried to sit up again. My hands and legs wouldn't stop shaking and I felt as if I might pass out any second. The nurse encouraged me to stand up, but as soon as I did the room began spinning and another wave of nausea hit. I knew we needed to get going so they could use the room, but there was just no way I could walk all the way out to the car. The nurse brought us a wheelchair and Jeff wheeled me out holding a little baggie just in case. Jeff was so sweet and careful on the drive back, avoiding all the bumps and taking it slow on all the turns.

He told me our RE had retrieved twenty-five eggs. I was amazed. I never thought we would get so many eggs. I knew the more eggs retrieved, the better our chances for fertilization, so twenty-five was wonderful news. We made it home and I crawled into bed to sleep some more. That night I started my Crinone, a vaginal progesterone suppository we would use through the first trimester of pregnancy if our cycle was successful.

Jen's Online Blog Entry

This day was very draining physically and mentally. We've done the best we can. It's up to our embies to grow now.

The next day our RE called with our fertilization results. Of the twenty-five eggs retrieved, only ten of them were mature enough to fertilize. Out of those ten, seven had fertilized and were growing at the lab. I'd be lying if I said I wasn't disappointed by the news. I had thought that with twenty-five eggs we would have around twelve fertilized eggs to work with. Instead we had seven, and I knew it was not likely that all seven would make it to Day 5 for our transfer. Jeff reminded me that he could have called with news that none of the eggs had fertilized. I immediately felt guilty for being disappointed. Jeff was right. I should be thrilled that we had seven little spuds, the pet name we gave our growing embryos. They were seven chances at a baby we never would have had otherwise. I said a prayer, thanking God for all he had done so far and waited along with Jeff for updates on our little spuds. I was still very sore from the retrieval and had a lot of bladder pain. I figured it would take a few days for me to feel back to myself and tried to ignore the discomfort.

Later that night, Jeff decided to go over to a friend's house for some time with "the guys." I knew he was under a lot of stress too and gladly sent him on his way. I did some stuff around the house but kept feeling worse and worse. Finally I decided to go to bed and sleep it off. I lay in bed tossing and turning. The bloating pain was much worse and my bladder pain was unrelenting. I scoured the medicine cabinet looking for something to bring relief. Of course I couldn't find a single antacid, Gas-X, or anything to help me feel better. I could not get the bloating to go away and nothing seemed to help. I walked around; I changed positions; I drank water. I was miserable and fed up with hurting all the time. I called Jeff and asked him to pick something up on his way home. By time Jeff arrived home I was in tears. I thankfully took the medicine Jeff had brought and finally fell asleep for the night.

Jen's Journal Entry 11-15-2000

I'm having terrible bloating today thanks to the retrieval yesterday. Everyday it's another pain. I got almost no sleep with terrible pain—I almost had to call it was so unbearable. Today seems better though. Sometimes I wonder if my grandma and grandpa are watching over me, helping when I feel I can't possibly continue. Strange thoughts, I suppose, but it's nice to think they're lending a hand to help us have a little one.

The second day after retrieval I was still not doing that great. My ovaries were still angry about the whole procedure they had been subjected to and I continued to feel extremely bloated. I brushed it off to the procedure and medication, trying to think only positive thoughts for our little spuds to keep growing. My mom decided to come in for a visit and I found myself struggling to keep our secret. Jeff had been such a wonderful support through our entire cycle, but I wanted so badly to share our journey with my mother. We were sitting on the couch when she asked me about still not feeling well and suggested I should make a doctor's appointment to get checked out. Rather than making up any more stories, I decided to let her in on our secret.

"Mom," I said. "I know why I haven't been feeling well." She quietly listened as I told her of our consult and our decision to attempt in vitro fertilization. I'm not really sure what reaction I was expecting, but she took the news in stride. She asked me about the procedure and what we had done so far. I proudly announced that we had seven embies growing right then but we wouldn't know for a couple more days how many would make it to transfer day. I explained why we had kept it a secret but that feeling sick for so long was wearing me down. She promised not to tell my dad or sister. We spent the rest of the day shopping together and then met Jeff for dinner.

All day I felt worse and worse. Neither the pain nor the bloating had improved. At dinner I pressed my hands against my pelvis in an attempt to ease some of the discomfort. I didn't want to spend the entire night complaining. I felt like I had been such a baby through most of our cycle. Usually I was a strong person who handled pain very well, but this in vitro cycle had pushed me to my limits. We talked about how our lives would change and what a child would mean to us. By the end of the day, I think my mom was much more excited and maybe even nervous about the path we were traveling. She had waited so long for us to have a baby. Even so, her biggest concern at the time was for her daughter who was not feeling so wonderful. She hugged me tightly before she left, telling me things would work out and to be strong.

Jen's Mom Remembers

Never will I forget the day on which my daughter told me that she and her husband had actually started the preliminaries for IVF. I knew how much they wanted a child and how sad and crushed they were after the loss of their first pregnancy, so I was overjoyed for them, but at that date could not help but worry because my daughter looked so sick. IVF, I knew, was conception outside the womb, but I had no idea how much had to be done beforehand to get to that point. So I was a little bit more reassured after my daughter explained to me what had been done to that point and what would still follow until she was actually pregnant. I thought, well—if her being so unwell is just the result of all this "prepping," I will have to accept that. Then, on my drive home, all of a sudden it hit me and I just knew without any doubt that everything would work out all right and that I would hold a little grandchild in my arms next year. With that conviction in my mind, my thoughts turned to baby showers, baby colors and baby gifts, and I could hardly keep from telling my husband when I got home. But I did keep mum and just told him that "some female problems" were the cause of our daughter's illness and that ended any further inquiry—thank God.

The third day after our retrieval our RE was due to call in another hour or two to update us on our little spuds. He informed us that of the seven little spuds we began with, we were down to three. He gave us our instructions for transfer day, which would be in a mere two days, and asked if we had any questions. I asked him about the symptoms I was having and was surprised to hear that I suffered from ovarian hyperstimulation syndrome (OHSS). Well, that definitely explained a lot. Here I thought I was just bloated from the procedure and come to find out fluid was building up in my abdomen. The OHSS explained the soreness, the pressure, and the bladder pain. I was instructed to monitor my urine output and to soak in a hot bath. Our doctor called in a prescription for Tylenol with Codeine to ease my pain and impressed upon me the importance of calling him the next day to let him know how I was feeling.

The Tylenol with Codeine did wonders for the pain. My chest was sore from shallow breathing and my urine output dropped to almost nothing, but I toughed it out at home. Our doctor was concerned that it might be better for my health if we delayed the transfer until my OHSS resolved. I was in tears at the thought of postponing our cycle.

Our Day 5 transfer was scheduled for Sunday, November 19, and somehow that turned out to be my best day. My pain had greatly diminished and I was determined to put our embies where they belonged: Inside their mommy.

Transfer day was very relaxed compared to retrieval day. I changed into my gown and Jeff and I both went into the room where the table and ultrasound machine were set up. We talked and joked with our RE, waiting for the embryologist to bring our two little guys we had decided to transfer. Suddenly, from the back of the lab we hear, "Cotter, right?" Jeff looked at me, I looked at him and we both looked at our doctor. "Yes!" we all yelled back. It was like hearing your stylist say "Oops!" while cutting your hair, or your mechanic mumbling, "Now where does this go?" as he fixes your brakes. For a split second that day my heart skipped a beat. The embryologist entered the room saying, "I was just making sure." I think there was an audible *whoosh* as we all let out our breath.

The transfer went smoothly. The procedure was similar to having a Pap smear done. There was only some pressure from the speculum and some mild discomfort when the fluid was injected. Jeff and I stared at our ultrasound picture of the injected fluid containing our two beautiful embryos (two Grade A blastocysts) as I lay on the cart for thirty minutes.

When the thirty minutes were up, I got dressed and hugged our RE before we left the clinic. He had done his best for us. Now it was up to our embies to implant. He told us that women who experience OHSS tend to produce very high quality embryos and often have a higher pregnancy rate because of this. That was a very reassuring thought to carry with us as we walked back to the car. Since I was finally feeling better, we decided to stop for lunch.

As we sat there talking about the transfer, I found myself looking at other couples seated in the restaurant. I wondered if any of them were celebrating a positive home pregnancy test, or discussing starting a family, or were in the midst of an in vitro cycle like us. When battling infertility, you tend to feel as if you are suffering all alone. None of our friends had trouble getting pregnant or understood what it was like to be in our shoes. Yet most likely at least one other couple having lunch that day understood our pain all too well.

Most of the lunch I spent smiling at Jeff, the man I loved more than anything on this earth for always loving me and putting up with my moods and tears the entire cycle. Jeff kept calling me Mom and I kept calling him Dad. The words seemed so strange to say. Could it really be possible? Could we really be lucky enough to bring a child into this world with the help of IVF? We would find out soon enough. We were both pleasantly surprised to learn that we did not have to wait a full two weeks for our pregnancy test (the beta hCG test) with a Day 5 transfer. Our first beta test was scheduled for November 25, only six days rather than the fourteen days we were anticipating. Later that night I lay in bed rubbing my belly and talking to our embies, praying for a gift from above.

I spent every one of those six days rubbing my belly and praying that at least one embryo would implant. Four days after our transfer, I felt a little sick to my stomach and experienced some mild cramping. I was very excited, thinking that these were the first signs of pregnancy, but in the back of my mind I knew they could also be the first signs of an oncoming menstrual cycle. I was still having some pain from my ovaries but physically I felt much better with the symptoms of my OHSS almost completely gone.

During those six days I found it difficult to focus on anything. I took those days off from work, thinking I would never be able to handle my period starting while working in an OB/GYN office. I also strongly felt I needed to be in a stress-free environment. No evidence existed to support the need for altering your physical activity post-transfer, but in my mind rest and relaxation would give us the best chance at a positive cycle. If I had learned anything from this experience, it was to listen closely to my inner voice.

Jen's Online Blog Entry

So many of our friends are pulling for us, I am thinking only positive thoughts for a good outcome. Thanks to all of our wonderful friends who constantly call to check up on me. I am determined to beat this syndrome and get back to a normal life. Jeff has been incredible, doing the shopping, cleaning, cooking—you name it. He has been on cloud 9 since the transfer and is convinced we're already pregnant. Just a few short days and this will all be over, but hopefully something truly wonderful will just be beginning.

Jeff's Online Blog Entry

I can't stop staring at the ultrasound picture showing the bright spot of fluid where our two embies are floating and waiting to attach.

The day of our first beta arrived and I awoke to feeling wonderful. No upset stomach. No ovarian pain. No cramping. Just a day like any other day. I couldn't help but feel a dark cloud form over my head. Jeff took the day off from work and sat quietly as our RE drew my blood. That one little vial of blood held all the answers. It would tell us either the happiest news of our lives or crush our hopeful hearts yet again. Jeff had been saying since transfer day that we were already pregnant, but even he seemed nervous as we walked out of the clinic, hand in hand.

We tried to enjoy the day as best as possible, but found ourselves watching the clock, waiting for that phone call. Those five hours felt like the longest five hours of my life. One o'clock came and went. Two o'clock came and went. I was getting further and further on edge, watching the hand go 'round and 'round while our phone sat silent. And yes, I admit it. I even lifted the receiver once just to make sure the phone was working. I was just about to lose my mind, thinking that our doctor must be calling all the couples with positive results first, when the phone finally rang just after three that afternoon. My hands shook as I answered.

Our RE greeted me and asked how I felt. We talked for a couple minutes and then he said, "Well, your hCG came back at 8." "Okay," I replied. "What does that mean?" "It means you're pregnant, Jen." My heart jumped into my chest and my voice quivered when I spoke. "Is 8 a good number?" I asked. He assured me that at six days post-transfer, he considered anything higher than 2 to be positive. Of course, he reminded me that it was still early and our next beta would tell us more. By now my heart was racing. I remember repeating, "Thank you, thank you" several times and agreed to come in for my second beta test in two days.

Jen's Journal Entry 11-25-2000

We are so excited but still a little worried until we get our second hCG on Monday. I'm so thrilled we're going to get to share our love and life with a child. Jeff is going to be a wonderful daddy and I'm going to do my best too. It seems our prayers have been answered and we're so thankful for that.

I hung up the phone and turned to Jeff. He seemed unsure if a beta hCG level of 8 was one to celebrate. I smiled at Jeff. "We're pregnant, Daddy!" Jeff's face lit up as he smiled. We hugged each other for a long time and said a prayer under our breaths for this wonderful gift. Five minutes later, I was on the phone with my mom to tell her the great news. She was extremely happy for us but, being the ever-protective mother, told me not to get too excited until our second beta. I asked if my dad was standing there, wondering what we were talking about. "No, he left the room. I told him you have been sick because of female problems so that he wouldn't ask too many questions. As I figured, it worked like a charm." I could almost see the smile on her face as she spoke.

Jeff called one of our closest friends and beamed with pride as he announced, "I'm going to be a dad!" We both wanted to share our wonderful news, but decided it would be best to only tell those friends we were closest to and who had followed our progress through our cycle. We both knew all too well that things could change very quickly. We could have a chemical pregnancy or we could lose the pregnancy. This was just one day out of many days ahead to make it to term with a healthy baby. But somehow our hearts refused to let our minds steal this blissful moment away from us. We were a mommy and a daddy at that moment and enjoyed it for the incredible blessing that it was.

Jen's Mom Remembers

I waited all morning for that darn phone to ring. Several times I picked up the phone to call my daughter but changed my mind. I did not want to add to her stress because of my impatience. When that call finally came, my heart was racing and I dropped the phone in my haste. How can you explain the emotions of utmost joy and happiness and at the same time the fear of something going wrong later? It was like I was afraid to be happy because I feared that so much might happen in the first three months.

Two days later we returned for our second beta test. I walked into the office all smiles as I passed through the doorway a pregnant woman rather than an infertile one. I felt as if my feet never touched the ground. I was having a queasy stomach on and off and my ovaries were once again reminding me of what they had gone through over the past few weeks. These were all wonderful annoyances to be dealing with. I was pregnant. But fate seemed determined to test our happiness when, two hours after my blood test, I started spotting. Jeff had taken another vacation day, but rather than going out as we had planned, we found ourselves snuggled in on the couch watching movies. Our anxiety grew as each time I got up to check, the spotting was worse. Could it really be over so quickly? Would we lose this pregnancy? I tried in vain to think about anything other than those heartbreaking questions.

I almost didn't want to answer the phone when it rang later that afternoon. I was scared to death that our RE would be on the other line with bad news. I picked up the phone to hear our doctor once again asking me how I was feeling. I told him that I had started spotting shortly after our blood work. "As you know," he began, "we look for a rise in your numbers. I would be happy to see your beta at 12-13." I forced myself to ask the question I had thought about all day. "What did my beta come back at?" He replied, "Your beta is 61."

The tears streamed down my face as he spoke those words. I dropped to my knees, trying not to cry into the phone. I vaguely remember him explaining many women experience spotting and bleeding early in pregnancy and that my numbers were very promising. I mumbled a thank you and hung up.

Jeff kneeled with me on the floor, not sure if my tears were of joy or sadness. "Our beta was 61, Daddy. We are definitely pregnant." Jeff broke down and we cried in each other's arms. All the stress and uncertainty of the day and our cycle came crashing down on us. I don't remember crying like that since losing our first pregnancy, but these were tears of joy that washed away four years of struggle and disappointment. We sat on the floor in each other's arms for a very long time, allowing tear after tear to run down our faces.

I not only cried in relief and happiness for the unborn child growing inside me, but also in acceptance for our first child, stolen before we ever shared a hug or a smile. My heart had been heavy for so many years but finally felt filled with love and joy as only a mother or mother-to-be understands. I don't know what all went through Jeff's mind as we sat there, but just as the heartache of losing our first pregnancy had brought us closer together, the beginning of this pregnancy entwined our souls even more.

I phoned my mother again with our good news. She seemed reluctant to get her hopes up but was very happy to hear my numbers had jumped so much. I knew things could still take a turn for the worse, but I was determined to enjoy every second of being pregnant. Holding back my emotions about the pregnancy wouldn't lessen the pain if something were to go wrong. I was a mommy-to-be and if it lasted for several weeks or several months, I was ecstatic to be given the chance once again.

Three days later I started to bleed. I woke up eleven days post-transfer to bright red blood and my heart sank. This can't be happening, I thought. To go from spotting to bright red bleeding couldn't be a good thing, and I worried we were having a miscarriage. I spoke with our RE and returned to his office for yet another beta test. I cried on the drive to his office, I cried on my way to work after the blood draw. I just couldn't take control of my emotions.

I left work and headed home. How could I think about anything except holding onto this baby? I was instructed to begin progesterone in oil injections 50 mg twice a day until the bleeding stopped. Since Crinone is a vaginal suppository and works more directly on the uterus, it wasn't possible to monitor my progesterone levels accurately through blood draws. By switching to the progesterone in oil (PIO) shots we would know exactly how much progesterone my body was getting.

The stipulation with our insurance coverage for the in vitro cycle was that we had to purchase all of our medications through a specific pharmacy. I called the pharmacy only to find out that they didn't have the PIO in stock and that it would take two to three days to get some. I relayed this information to our RE and he firmly said, "Find the PIO somewhere else. You need to start it today."

I called Jeff at work sobbing. I couldn't take the stress and searching for the PIO was the last straw. I felt as if I was being punished. Why was this happening? Why couldn't I just be like everyone else: get pregnant on my own, have a positive home pregnancy test, and go on to have an uneventful pregnancy. Was it really that much to ask? Hadn't I been through enough already?

I called one pharmacy, then another, and another. No one had the PIO in stock. The day just kept getting worse. I called Jeff again and asked him to please come home. I needed his strength to keep me from falling apart. During his drive home I finally found a pharmacy that had the capabilities of mixing their own formulas and could have the PIO ready in thirty minutes. Jeff wrapped his arms around me as soon as he walked through the door and calmed my nerves, assuring me it would be okay and that things would work out. We got to the pharmacy, bought our PIO, and made it back home in time for Jeff to give me my first PIO injection before heading back to work after an extended lunch.

The progesterone in oil shot was extremely painful. It was a thick solution and difficult to push through the needle, and worse yet it had to be given into the muscle. A large bump formed at the injection site and was still hurting later that night. Our doctor called with my third beta results. He said he would be happy with a beta level of 150 for progression of a normal pregnancy or a little less if I was possibly miscarrying a twin.

My hCG was 237. I was shocked. I honestly thought my number would be lower and that we would be losing our second pregnancy. Our first ultrasound was scheduled for December 7, a whole seven days away. Those seven days were more stressful than the six days following our transfer.

I ended up having the bright red bleeding for one day only and then continued to spot for two days after that. I ended up getting four PIO shots, and they gave me a whole new perspective on what other women endured. I had two lumps form at the injection sites that lasted for almost a week. They were painful enough to wake me in the night if I happened to roll over on them. I was very happy to return to using the Crinone when the spotting stopped.

Jeff and I found ourselves back in the office December 7, holding hands tightly as our RE placed the vaginal ultrasound probe. Much to our delight, a large dark area appeared on the screen immediately. I was five weeks pregnant and we were seeing the gestational sac just as expected. I had been feeling pretty nauseous over the past four days and was convinced we had two little stinkers inside causing havoc. Our RE was only able to locate one sac, though. Of course, twins would have been wonderful but Jeff and I knew one child would be much more manageable. We couldn't ask for anything more than a single, healthy baby after all these years.

Our second ultrasound was on December 13, 2000. We held hands tightly again, hoping to see progression in the pregnancy. Much to our surprise, we not only saw the beginnings of our child but also heard its heartbeat. Jeff wiped tears from his eyes as we listened to swooshing at 140 beats per minute. I will never forget that day. Were we out of the woods? By no means. But we both felt as if we had some breathing room now and could relax just a little. At my second ultrasound I was six weeks, one day pregnant with a due date of August 8, 2001 and was already having significant nausea on a nightly basis. But I vowed not to complain. Any symptom of pregnancy was welcomed. I must say, how quickly things would change.

Our third and final ultrasound with our RE was on December 22, 2000. Once again, we listened to the swooshing of our baby's heart, soothing us at 140 beats per minute. I was very excited that our next appointment would be with an obstetrician. Yet part of me was very sad to be saying goodbye to our RE. He had taken such good care of us and had given us the child we never thought we would have. He had called with every lab result, answered every question, given support when we were feeling lost. I hugged him before we left and thanked him. No words could ever really say enough but somehow I knew he understood the weight of those two simple words. We told our RE we would come back for a visit as parents.

Chapter Three

Waddling on the Other Side of Infertility

At seven weeks gestation my nausea suddenly began lingering from morning until night. I felt very tired but still kept up with life fairly well. Although we originally planned on celebrating Christmas with my family at our home, I was starting to think that might not work so well after all. Cooking had become more and more of a challenge. I couldn't stand the smell or feel of raw meat. How in the world would I ever be able to fix Christmas dinner? I spoke with my mom and asked her if we could move the celebration to their house. She was more than willing to help out her sick, pregnant daughter. At this point my dad hadn't asked too many questions, but he expressed concern that I was still sick enough to change our Christmas plans. I decided the time had come to tell my dad and sister about our special Christmas present from Santa.

My dad listened as I told him my "female problem" meant that I was pregnant. "Oh really," were his first words. My dad—always the quiet one in the family. My sister's response was quite different. She squealed into the phone and started crying. She had pretty much given up hope that we would ever have a baby and had come to accept that she would never be called Auntie. She was very surprised to find out we had done in vitro and kept it a secret. I wasn't feeling well at all, but Christmas was going to be very special for everyone.

By Christmas eve my nights were pretty bad. Just the smell of food was enough to make my stomach turn and nothing tasted good. The rash I developed at the beginning of our cycle was getting worse. Red, itchy bumps stretched across my lower back and elbows. I already had a lovely green look to me, almost like those poor people you see hanging over the railing of a boat, battling motion sickness.

My mom had a gift for the baby already and couldn't wait for me to open it. Inside was a cute little pink bug that squeaked. I smiled at my mom, knowing she was thinking the same as me: If there was any truth to the old wives' tale of having rotten sickness while pregnant with a girl, I should be buying lots of pink. Later that night, as we sat talking, she told me how much she hoped I would have a daughter to share all those special moments she had shared with me. I had wanted a little girl from the start, too. I dreamed of shopping trips and helping her with her hair, but I continued to call our unborn child "little peanut." Jeff and I decided we wouldn't find out the sex of the baby. Since our in vitro cycle had been so planned and coordinated, we wanted something to be a surprise.

Jen's Mom Remembers

I truly believe this: during a daughter's pregnancy, we mothers become "extra sensory perceptive" individuals. I knew I could tune into my daughters' emotions, fears and feelings without a single word being said. During the entire time of their pregnancies, I shared an unbelievable closeness with both of my daughters that came to an ultimate high at the time of them giving birth. Perhaps it is the time in their life that they need their mother the most, to lean on, to inquire from and to be reassured. After all, how can a man, no matter how loving and caring, tell them from experience what is going on with their body and mind during the nine months of growing a child inside? I have shared the ups and downs during my daughter's pregnancy fully—to that my phone bill can attest. But I would not have wanted it any other way. Perhaps being so close during that time, we are in turn preparing for the wonderful job of a grandmother.

Christmas day found us at Jeff's parents' house with his parents and one of his brothers. We planned to give special gifts to Jeff's parents to announce our exciting news. I had placed a poem in a silver picture frame and we had bought Jeff's dad a grandpa sweatshirt. We thought it would be fun to have Jeff's parents open the gifts simultaneously when we sat around the tree. But on the drive over, Jeff was too excited about sharing the news and wanted to give them their gifts right away. That was fine with me. Then I wouldn't have to make more excuses about not eating much for dinner. When we arrived, Jeff's brother wasn't there yet, but Jeff just couldn't wait. Rather than giving them both their gifts, we had them both open the picture frame.

The poem, "A Special Gift" read:

Although I am very, very small here inside,
I asked Mommy and Daddy to share the surprise
On this wonderful blessed Christmas Day,
To let Grandma and Grandpa know that I'm on the way.

This precious frame is my gift to you,
To hold my photo when I am brand new.
August is still a long ways away,
But until then I'll just say, "Have a very Happy Holiday."

Jeff's parents were stunned and very happy for us. His brother arrived shortly after and we announced he was going to be an uncle again. The rest of the day went well and late in the evening we packed up for the hour-long drive home. Right before walking out the door, I went to the bathroom and discovered bright red bleeding again. I closed my eyes, sighed and left the house without saying a word to anyone about it. By the time we arrived home I had bled quite a bit, but the bleeding stopped by the next morning. Apparently our roller-coaster ride was far from over.

The first trimester of my pregnancy was difficult, to say the least. I started vomiting at around eight and a half weeks. The vomiting occurred initially at nighttime, usually starting around four in the afternoon. Almost every night after work, Jeff walked through the door to find me slouched over the toilet, tossing my cookies. I would be retching and crying, unable to stop either. If I ate food, I threw up. If I drank liquids, I threw up. If I didn't eat or drink, I threw up. The barking dog made me vomit; standing up too quickly made me sick. I couldn't watch television anymore because the movement on screen would set off the vomiting and I couldn't work on the computer for more than thirty minutes at a time because that made me nauseous. I was emotionally and physically drained. Jeff rubbed my back, held my hair and told me to hang in there. So many times I told him I couldn't make it. There was just no way I could survive until my due date of August 8, 2001.

I had such deep retching that my stomach and back ached for hours and my nose burned. Jeff kidded around, asking me if I was ready for number two as I heaved yet again. I knew he was trying to help, but I couldn't smile. My pregnancy sickness was a sickness unlike any I had felt before. Take the worst flu you've ever had and the worst hangover you've ever had and multiply them by a thousand. I could barely ride in the car. The Sea-bands I bought didn't help much. The exhaust from passing cars and trucks also turned my stomach, even with the car windows closed. I had to stay out of the kitchen when Jeff cooked; the sight and smell of food was too much. People actually joked with me about how green I looked all the time. After a really difficult day, I phoned my obstetrician asking for help. I was to the point I couldn't even keep water down anymore. I was only nine weeks along and the second trimester wasn't coming any time soon.

A home nurse was scheduled to come to the house the next day to start an IV. Most likely I was dehydrated and would feel better with some fluids. When she arrived she started explaining about the Reglan pump I would use. The pump was a small device that would deliver Reglan (a medication to prevent nausea and vomiting) through a catheter into my body. I thought my OB had changed his mind and decided to start medication rather than fluids. The nurse inserted a tiny catheter into my thigh. The catheter was then attached to the pump. The pump would slowly dose me with the Reglan throughout the day and night. I would wear it twenty-four hours a day, covering it with plastic when I took a shower. Every so often, I would need to change the needle to protect against infection and change the medication reservoir when it reached a certain low level. By time the nurse left I was already getting some relief from the medication.

Part of the training that afternoon included other ways of lessening the nausea and vomiting without medication. Every suggestion the home nurse made pointed to something I was doing in error. I was supposed to avoid gas-causing foods, not drink from a straw, and keep something in my stomach at all times with snacking throughout the day. I was also supposed to eat something before getting out of bed each morning. As I sat there feeling better, I worried about the baby. Every medication carries risk during pregnancy and although Reglan has been used in pregnant mice with no ill effects to the fetus, there weren't adequate human studies for obvious reasons. Up to this point I hadn't even taken Tylenol for pain and I felt uncomfortable taking the Reglan.

I had only been on the medication for four hours when I pulled the small catheter from my thigh. Most people may not understand my actions. I had finally found some relief and I was choosing to suffer instead. But we had gone through so much to get pregnant. I would never forgive myself if the baby was born with problems because of the medication. I chose my baby's health over my own comfort. I felt if I followed the other guidelines about lessening the nausea and vomiting, that I could manage. I was already learning what other mothers know all too well: You sacrifice yourself for the benefit of your children.

The rest of the night went well but the nausea and vomiting returned the next day. Jeff arrived home, loaded down with snack foods like crackers, cereal bars, fruit cups and peppermint candies. I ate so many peppermint candies I was half expecting to see red and white stripes on my face when I looked in the mirror. To this day, I still cannot bring myself to taste another peppermint candy. I hit my lifetime limit in those difficult weeks of my first trimester.

After the home nurse's visit, some days were tolerable with only nausea. Some days were unbearable with nausea all day long and vomiting for several hours at night. Jeff was always comforting and supportive, reminding me again and again that I could make it through the pregnancy. At thirteen weeks, the vomiting slowly subsided and I was left with only the nausea. At fifteen weeks my nausea was disappearing and I was able to eat an actual meal rather than just snack. Just before I hit sixteen weeks, I got food poisoning. I had one more night of terrible vomiting and then my stomach finally settled down.

I was also faced with bleeding issues during the first trimester. On two separate occasions we went rushing to the office for an ultrasound when I had large amounts of bright red bleeding. The second bleeding episode occurred while I had the flu and had been coughing and sneezing all day long. Much to our relief, the baby was doing well with a strong heartbeat. The ultrasound did show that the placenta was somewhat low. That, combined with the constant coughing, was likely causing me to bleed. I used saline nose spray, Breathe Right strips and slept a lot during the flu. I just didn't have the energy or the desire to do much else. I probably saw every episode of *A Baby Story* that week. Watching the joy of other couples giving birth to their baby helped me get through a very difficult week. Thankfully, once I was over the flu the bleeding stopped.

I have looked back through my IVF cycle journal as I write this book and smile at the words I wrote so easily: *I will not complain. I welcome every symptom of pregnancy.* The first trimester of pregnancy really took the wind out of my sails. I so looked forward to being a pregnant woman but, rather than experiencing all the joys and excitement most women experience, I was pummeled with bleeding problems, the flu, food poisoning and severe nausea and vomiting. My rash continued to worsen. It spread across my back, my elbows, my legs, my vulva and my stomach. No amount of scratching could satisfy that itch. I often scratched to the point of bleeding and then scratched some more. My skin turned dark red and purple where the skin opened. I applied an antibacterial ointment to protect against infection but otherwise simply tried my best not to scratch all day long. My OB questioned if a progesterone allergy was the cause of my severe nausea, vomiting and the unusual rash. He also questioned whether I might have a diseased gallbladder. Labs to check for a diseased gallbladder all came back normal and a progesterone allergy was never proven. Apparently I was just one of those unlucky women experiencing a difficult pregnancy.

As I struggled during the worst weeks, I uttered four words to Jeff that will haunt me forever. "I hate being pregnant." I have such guilt for saying those words. Pregnancy was something I had prayed and worked so hard for, yet what at first seemed like such a blessing had come to feel like a curse. Our IVF cycle had been very hard on me physically and I felt even more drained after the first trimester. During the first trimester, I gained a lot of weight by snacking all day long. I looked much further along than I really was and I already worried about losing the extra pounds once the baby arrived. There really is truth in the saying, "That which doesn't kill you will only make you stronger." I had survived the first trimester and was finally starting to feel human again. I had a nice round belly already and would often stop as I passed a mirror to rub it. I couldn't help but smile, knowing that our baby was under my shirt rather than a pillow.

The world became a wonderful place once again during the second trimester. I was able to eat a full meal, take the dog for walks, plant flowers in the garden, live life rather than watch it pass by from the couch. We shopped for furniture, a stroller and a rocker. One day while shopping Jeff and I found ourselves standing in the baby section of a department store. I was obviously pregnant and in the right spot, yet I felt strange standing there, touching the tiny socks and shirts. I kept thinking; *This is a dream and soon I'm going to wake up lying next to Jeff with a flat stomach and an empty feeling inside.* I leaned over to Jeff and whispered, "Do you feel out of place?" He smiled back, nodding his head.

We found a cute little outfit that would work for a boy or a girl, but I hesitated as we headed up to pay. Buying our first baby item together was a moment to cherish forever. Clothing, not for a friend or relative's baby, but for our own child. The realization of that hit me and I almost placed the outfit back among the others. Jeff noticed and asked if I had changed my mind for something else. "No," I said. "But what if..." Jeff stopped me before I could finish. He took my hand and reassured me. "It's okay, Jenifer. We're all going to do just fine."

Did I really believe buying that outfit would jinx our pregnancy? No. But living with infertility for so many years, I allowed my skin to thicken as a means of dealing with all the pain and disappointment. It changed my outlook on everything. I should have been enjoying this incredible miracle, but instead I was still waiting for it to be stolen from us. I reminded myself I had vowed to enjoy every second that I possibly could and I let the "what if" fade to the back of my mind for good.

We started transforming the second bedroom into a nursery soon after that. I was excited to get started before my belly got in the way. We washed the walls in pastel yellow and blue. I painted fluffy white clouds on the ceiling and hand painted nursery rhyme images on the walls. It was about then that I felt the first movements of our little peanut.

I was sixteen weeks pregnant, lying in bed before starting the day, when I felt the faintest twinge deep inside my belly. The first twinge I brushed off as my imagination. By the third twinge I couldn't stop smiling. I lay there for another thirty minutes rubbing my belly, talking to my child and savoring that special moment before running to the phone to share my exciting news with Jeff. I spent the next two weeks waiting for that feeling of movement again, but nothing. At eighteen weeks I found myself sitting on the floor of the nursery petting our dog as her head lay across my expanding belly. Jeff was diligently hammering the trim along the wall when little peanut rolled in my tummy. I squealed with delight. Sure enough, a couple minutes later the baby rolled again, then again, then again. There are no words to describe the sensation of our baby moving inside my belly. Those movements brought such a flood of emotions. I was no longer simply pregnant, but nurturing a small life inside me.

Jeff's hammering had apparently sparked our little peanut, because from that day on I was overjoyed to feel movement throughout the day and night. The twinges and rolls soon turned into kicks, pokes and punches. I spent hours in the nursery, softly singing as the rocker glided back and forth. I enjoyed those quiet moments with my unborn child, bonding with little peanut before our eyes had ever met. It was such an incredible feeling that I couldn't wait for Jeff to feel the kicks too. Each night and each morning Jeff lay with his hand on my belly. It became a ritual for us. Usually the baby moved and I'd smile at Jeff. "Did you feel that?" I would ask and Jeff would sigh, "No."

One morning was quite different, though. Jeff had just returned from a business trip and was poky getting up that morning. Like every morning for the past few months, his hand gently rested on my belly. Suddenly, I felt a hard kick. Jeff's eyes opened and he looked at me. "Was that a kick?" "Yes, Daddy. That's your child saying good morning." I smiled. Jeff was amazed as he felt another kick and then another. It was one memory of our pregnancy I hope to never forget. The intense love in Jeff's eyes as he felt his child move for the first time filled my heart with joy. He rolled over to face me and lay there for twenty minutes, feeling kick after kick. Finally, little peanut drifted off to sleep and Jeff decided he had better head out to work. He kissed my belly before leaving that morning with such gentleness, I almost cried.

The second trimester really was the honeymoon phase for us. With the nausea, vomiting and bleeding problems behind us, we fully enjoyed being pregnant. Slowly, the nursery filled with soft toys, blankets and tiny clothes. Each night Jeff would read to our child as I rubbed my belly. Even then Jeff's voice would incite movement, as if little peanut knew it was Daddy's voice talking about green eggs and ham. I was greeted with smiles from most everyone I passed. My green color faded and I began to glow. I had more energy than I had had for quite some time and enjoyed shopping for all those baby items I never thought would fill our home. Although Jeff and I had been determined not to find out the sex of our child, feeling the baby move changed our minds. We were already bonding so closely with little peanut and wanted to learn more about the little life impacting ours so deeply. I had always hoped for a girl but started having dreams of a little boy with dark hair. Jeff had said he would love to have a little girl as well, but I had a sneaking suspicion he was really hoping for a boy. So, our resolve faded and we asked to know the sex of our child at our next ultrasound.

Our baby was growing fast, measuring two weeks ahead of our estimated due date by ultrasound. And, as luck would have it, the baby had its legs crossed throughout the ultrasound. Jeff and I were both a little disappointed, but enjoyed watching our little peanut squirm on the screen. Everything looked completely normal except for the baby's stomach. My obstetrician had been unable to locate the gastric bubble on our previous ultrasound and was unable to locate it again (normally there is a small bubble of air in the stomach). We were concerned we had not seen the air bubble, so we were referred to a perinatologist for a more detailed ultrasound.

The days leading up to our appointment with the perinatologist dragged by. I vowed not to worry, but who was I kidding? It seemed our strength was being tested yet again. Unfortunately for Jeff, he had a meeting the day of our ultrasound, but luckily my mom was able to join me.

As soon as we entered the room, I explained to the doctor that we wanted to find out the sex of the baby but I did not want him to tell my mother or me. I asked him to please write the sex of the baby on a piece of paper and seal it in an envelope so that Jeff would be the first to know. Both the doctor and the nurse smiled at my request and assured me that they wouldn't spoil the surprise. The perinatologist found the gastric bubble immediately. I let out a sigh of relief and was able to relax and enjoy our beautiful baby on the screen. When the doctor showed us the baby's profile my mom exclaimed, "He has Jeff's nose!" My mom felt strongly that I had a little boy kicking away inside. I was already twenty-six weeks along and every organ was developed and looked normal. I was very relieved to hear our baby was doing wonderfully and that we shouldn't worry.

As my mother and I walked down the hospital hallway, she held up the envelope to peek at the writing inside. Much to her dismay, the nurse had folded the paper in half for added security. She would have to wait until later that night, just like the rest of us. I couldn't help but smile at my mom's curiosity. It was killing her not to know and I promised she would be the first phone call we made once Jeff got home.

Jeff Remembers

I was at work when Jen and her mom were at the doctor's office. Jen was nice enough to have the nurse seal the surprise in an envelope so neither Jen nor her mom knew what it said. After work, I walked into the house and there stood Jen with the envelope in her hand. She said she didn't know what it said. I didn't believe her at first. I held the envelope up to the light to cheat a little and I thought I saw the word boy. I got very excited at that moment and ripped it open. "Boy!" the little memo said. I smiled and said, "I'm going to have a son!" I gave Jen a huge hug and thanked her for letting me be the first to know.

Standing with the envelope in my hand when Jeff walked through the door reminded me of the excitement I had that day surprising him about our first pregnancy. As Jeff ripped open the envelope and peeked at the note inside, I knew it was a boy before he ever spoke a word. His smile and the sparkle in his eyes said it all. My dreams of a little boy with dark hair were soon to come true.

Jeff asked me if I was disappointed to learn we would have a son. I could honestly say that I was not. Although I had always talked about wanting a little girl, deep down I was very excited to have a little boy. Apparently, Jeff had hoped for a boy all along but was afraid to say anything and upset me, thinking I was so excited about a little girl. Funny how sometimes you don't really know what it is in life you want until you've received a gift that touches your heart so deeply.

I immediately called my parents and relayed the happy news. My mom's first words were, "I knew it!" We called more family and friends to share the newest Cotter Clan development. That night while lying in bed, Jeff kept whispering, "That's my boy," as our son kicked and punched my belly. We tucked the envelope away along with the ultrasound pictures and slept a peaceful night's sleep.

Jen's Mom Remembers

The trip to the specialist was a stressful event. The fear that something was wrong was on my mind but even so I kept reassuring my daughter. The moment an 'all okay' was given, all that stress vanished. I could tell from the expression on the physician's face while he was looking at the ultrasound that he knew immediately what sex the baby was. Just then he rotated the picture and I could see an outline by the leg that a little girl would not have, so it was no surprise to learn of a little boy coming our way.

Having made it through the worries of a problem with our baby's development, it was sure to be smooth sailing from then on. But at the risk of sounding like a broken record, how quickly things would change once again. As the end of the second trimester approached, my nausea and vomiting returned. Although it wasn't as severe as the first trimester, it was very painful to retch with a pregnant belly. I could hardly stand the sight of saltine crackers or peppermint candies, so I usually ate breakfast and something small for lunch and then lived on chocolate milk shakes for dinner. For whatever reason, milk shakes seemed to be the one thing my stomach approved of after three in the afternoon and who was I to say otherwise? We were two-thirds of the way through our pregnancy, we had the nursery finished for the most part, and we were still glowing over the news of having a baby boy.

During the third trimester of pregnancy, we decided upon a name for our son. We had always liked the name Nicholas, and it was one of the few names we both agreed on. I had asked Saint Nick for a special present at Christmas, and he had delivered indeed. Nicholas is also a prominent name in both the Irish and German traditions, our family's strongest heritage. The name has come to fit him perfectly.

The glory days of the second trimester slowly faded and were replaced with days filled with Braxton Hicks contractions (false labor pains) and nights filled with unbelievable hip and back pain. I proudly displayed a very large belly and my body ached everywhere. I was, however, excited to finally have our professional pregnancy photos taken. For the most part, I had not worn pregnancy very well. I always received such nice compliments from friends and family and even strangers, but I felt anything but beautiful or radiant. Having gone through so much to become pregnant and having dealt with so many rough days and nights since our first beta, I wanted something to remind me of

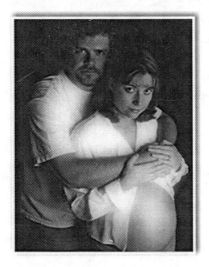

the good moments. A local professional photographer arrived at our home midway through the third trimester. I had coaxed Jeff into being in the pictures as well. After all, we had done everything as a couple and it was that strength and love that carried us through. I wanted to have a snapshot of a moment in time, the expecting parents waiting for a very special delivery.

I must say, I was not optimistic that the pictures would be anything spectacular. Not that I doubted our photographer's talent, but when I looked in the mirror I saw a tired, sore, pale woman—not exactly the ideal model for a photo shoot. I still remember asking Jeff if he thought my belly was big enough to look good in the pictures. He laughed. When we received the proofs in the mail a few weeks later, I understood why.

Our photographer had done the impossible. She had captured the love between Jeff, me and our unborn child, and

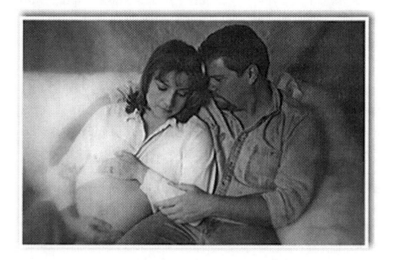

somehow had found the beauty of pregnancy that I couldn't see. The smooth skin of my belly reflected the light and the smiles on our faces spoke of our undeniable innocence about what becoming a parent really entailed. Our pregnancy photos are one of my most treasured possessions. When I look at them I only remember the good moments: hearing the heartbeat for the first time; watching little peanut squirm across the ultrasound screen; learning we were having a boy; witnessing wave after wave of movement across my belly. The pictures of Jeff and I together are priceless. They speak of the tenderness in the man I love and his role as my protector and supporter.

Near the end of the third trimester, we had our one and only baby shower. Much to the disappointment of family and friends, I begged them to have a single, small shower for me. The nausea and vomiting were difficult to deal with and the thought of a large gathering was too overwhelming. Our house was filled with gifts and well wishes. So many of our guests never thought they would celebrate such a wonderful day with us, but we fooled them all. It was a warm, sunny day in June, with the birds singing and the flowers blooming; a perfect day to celebrate the start of something new.

My belly continued to measure ahead (bigger than expected) throughout the third trimester and I held on to the hope that either Nicholas would make an early entrance into the world or my OB would take pity on my poor body and induce me before Nicholas grew too large for me to deliver easily. The summer heat left me trapped in the house once again. With false labor pains occurring often, we missed social gatherings. Several times I found myself counting contractions every five minutes, but they were of low intensity. I would walk through the house at night to ease my back and hip pain and to encourage my false labor to become true, but to no avail. Nicholas would arrive when he was ready and not a moment before, regardless of my walking or gentle hinting that he would have a lot more room to stretch if he was on the outside.

Jen's Journal Entry 5-28-2001

The reality is starting to sink in. Most of the time I am thrilled and excited, and then other times I'm nervous and anxious. Not so much about the delivery, but just the incredible change about to happen in our lives.

By thirty-seven weeks I was on a bland diet that consisted mainly of chocolate milk shakes and back to crying at night when the hip pain and vomiting became overwhelming. My skin was beefy red and purple from the rash and refused to clear up, even with antibiotics.

The day of my thirty-seven week checkup, I felt horrible. I was so nauseous; I couldn't bring myself to eat any breakfast. It also seemed that Nicholas was more quiet than usual, which worried me a little. I arrived at the office, feeling even worse. My blood pressure was elevated for the first time and the nurses commented on my pale appearance. My OB had an uneasy feeling about the way I looked and was concerned about my elevated blood pressure and fluid retention. My cervix was dilated to one centimeter and was already beginning to thin out. With my symptoms and a favorable cervix, we decided I should be admitted to the hospital for induction of labor.

I called Jeff from the office to let him know about the plan, much to his disbelief. He was at the tail end of a huge project at work and had jokingly forbidden me to go into labor until the following week, when he would be finished with the project. His exact words were, "Are you serious? We're having the baby now?" I explained that I was most definitely serious and that we all felt it was best to induce me with the way I was feeling. I could very easily just be having a bad day or it could be the first signs of preeclampsia.

I was shooed out of the office with smiles and hugs for good luck. We had packed my bag a few weeks earlier, so I spent some time with our dog while waiting for Jeff to arrive home. Soon we were on our way to the hospital to have our baby. I was admitted for a slow Pitocin induction. The Pitocin was started around noon and by half past one, I was in a regular contraction pattern.

I called my parents to let them know we were in the hospital and that we should be holding our son within the next one to two days. My parents excitedly stated that they were on their way and would stay overnight at our house to watch our dog and be close by should anything happen.

At the hospital, the IV fluids eased my nausea and made me feel better almost immediately. My blood pressure was back to normal as well. Jeff and I sat smiling at each other, both a little amazed that we were actually in the hospital about to have a baby. Jeff informed me that he was going to suffer right along with me. If I couldn't eat, then he wouldn't eat. If I was up all night, then he would stay up all night. It was a very sweet gesture on his part but short-lived when his stomach started growling two hours later.

While Jeff made a run to the cafeteria, my OB stopped in. He said his plan was to do a very slow induction, allow me to contract through the night and then break my water in the morning. Ten minutes after the doctor left the room, Jeff walked back in with a cheeseburger and fries which smelled delicious. With feeling so sick, I hadn't eaten all day and wasn't allowed anything while being induced. Jeff was nice enough to tease me by waving the smell over my way. It was all in good fun. I gave him my best puppy dog eyes and convinced him it would be okay if I had just a couple fries. And let me just say, they were some pretty incredible fries.

Two hours later my parents stopped to visit before heading to our place. My contractions were becoming much more intense by then but still manageable. Shortly after my parents left, I decided to soak in the Jacuzzi to help ease some of the pain. The warm, bubbly water stimulated my contractions quite a bit, and actually made them much more tolerable. Unfortunately, there wasn't room in the Jacuzzi for Jeff, so he was stuck kneeling next to the tub, holding my hand.

Soon I was back in bed and contracting regularly. I wanted to hold off on medication as long as possible because I wanted to experience as much of labor as I could tolerate. By half past seven, the contractions were extremely painful and I called the nurse for some medication. I was surprised after such good contractions to still be only dilated one centimeter, the same as in the office earlier that day. I was given Nubain through my IV, which gives pain relief for approximately four hours. I still felt the contractions, but they were much more subdued. My OB continued to increase my Pitocin slowly over the next several hours.

Jeff and I watched television to pass the time and talked about everyday things. We watched my contractions peak and he helped me relax through them as much as possible. By eleven, Jeff drifted off to sleep. I hoped to catch a few hours of sleep myself, but my brain refused to shut down. By one in the morning, the pain grew very intense again. I held off on medication, hoping that the intense contractions would dilate my cervix more so I would be able to receive an epidural.

Jeff awoke to me softly crying around three A.M. when I was breathing through a very painful contraction. He sat next to me on the bed and rubbed my feet. I reached the point where I couldn't lie still anymore. I finally decided to call the nurse to check me to see if I was dilated enough for an epidural. Once again, I was disappointed to hear her say I was only dilated two centimeters. The only good news was that I was almost completely effaced, meaning my cervix had thinned out. Now I just needed to dilate to ten centimeters and we would be ready to start pushing. Ten centimeters seemed a lifetime away at the rate I was going. Since I was undergoing Pitocin induction, the contractions were much more intense than unassisted labor. Because my cervix was both dilating and thinning, I was offered an epidural and jumped at the chance. Without an induction, I would not have received my epidural so early for fear of slowing or stopping my labor. There was no risk of this happening since the Pitocin would continue to stimulate my contractions.

At four A.M., the anesthesiologist arrived. To sit slouched over with a huge pregnant belly and painful contractions was difficult, but to go without an epidural was out of the question while being induced. Insertion of the needle into the space around the spinal cord should not be painful, but the first needle was very painful, so the anesthesiologist had to remove it and try a second time. The second time was uncomfortable but not painful, so he taped the catheter in place. Ten minutes later I vomited rather violently, something that can occur following insertion of the epidural. However, with the epidural in place, my pain subsided within a few minutes and was completely gone within a half-hour. Now I would be able to get some much needed rest, or so I thought.

At 4:30 A.M., my water broke. The nurse checked me once again and of course I was still dilated two centimeters. She helped me change gowns and freshened up the bed. Shortly after my water broke, our little peanut's heart rate started to dip. I changed position and the heart rate recovered nicely. Several minutes later it dipped again. Because our baby was not tolerating the Pitocin very well, the drip was turned off. I changed position to lie on my left side and Nicholas did well from then on.

By 6:00 A.M., I was having extremely painful contractions on the right side. I tried to tough them out, but they were too much to bear. I called the nurse and asked that the anesthesiologist come re-dose my epidural. At 6:30 A.M., I became violently ill again with intense heaving and profound vomiting up through my nose. At that point I broke down and started sobbing. I was exhausted and tired of being so sick all of the time. It was shift change for the nurses and my new nurse came in shortly after to clean me up. She gently caressed my hair and offered words of encouragement. I appreciated her efforts, but I was suffering and wanted this to be over. I had spent the last hour worrying that I would end up with a C-section. If I didn't deliver within twenty-four hours of my water breaking, they would take me for a C-section. Once the Pitocin was turned off, my contractions decreased significantly. I knew the clock was ticking and we had to be careful with the Pitocin since little peanut had already shown his dislike of the induction. Jeff held me as I cried, trying to ease my worries and pain. My new nurse decided to check my cervix even though it had only been two and a half hours since my last check.

She shocked us both when she announced I was completely dilated and the baby's head was already down. Once I lay on my back for a few minutes, I could feel the head sitting there. I had dilated very quickly (8 cm in 2.5 hours) and it had likely triggered my vomiting. She hurried off to phone our OB, telling me, "No matter what, don't push!" Yeah—easy for her to say. Just then the anesthesiologist arrived to re-dose my epidural. Soon the room was buzzing with activity as the nurses prepared for the arrival of our baby. I was so excited to almost be at the point of pushing.

Resisting the urge to push, I focused on anything and everything around me. I told Jeff our OB better arrive soon or a nurse would be delivering our son. Our OB arrived by 7:45 A.M. and quickly gloved up. I finally got the green light to start pushing. I pushed three times and Nicholas' head crowned. Jeff was amazed to look down and see dark hair. Three more pushes and his head was out. One more push and Nicholas entered the world with a hearty cry. He christened our OB and two of the nurses with tinkles as he was lifted to rest on my belly. He was the most beautiful baby I had ever seen. His head was perfectly shaped and he was absolutely gorgeous. The proud daddy cut the cord and smiled up at me. Jeff had tears in his eyes and seemed pretty shaken up over the intense excitement of our son's birth. He never left Nicholas' side from the time he was born. He gently touched his child and was overjoyed when Nick's tiny hand encircled his finger.

He followed Nicholas over to the warmer, snapping pictures. The scene was so heart-warming: the new daddy carefully checked his son over and spoke softly to him. Suddenly, Jeff was back at my side, bending to kiss me. He apologized for walking away. I told him to not be silly and go back to his son. After all, I wasn't going anywhere.

Jeff Remembers

On the morning of July 20, 2001 with 18 hours of labor and an epidural behind us (well, Jen, I guess), it was time to bring Nick into the world. When the nurse checked Jen she was dilated and Nick was already crowning. Immediately, the nurses started to get prepped and pages were sent to get the doctor in the room before Jen had the baby. Once he entered the room, Jen gave a few pushes and I saw dark hair. I remember the doctor saying this won't work and out came the scissors and "snip." At that moment I learned what episiotomy means. Within minutes and a few pushes, Nick was born. I cut the cord and followed him to the warmer where the nurse cleaned him up. I started taking pictures and just stared at this beautiful baby boy. I had tears of joy running down my cheeks. I suddenly realized I had forgotten about Jen. I embraced her with all the love in the world and handed her Nick to hold.

Every single moment of our journey to parenthood, whether good or bad, was worth the incredible feeling of finally having a child all our own. Nicholas' cry was such sweet music. I just couldn't stop smiling. Jeff carried the tiny bundle over to our OB so that he could hold the little miracle he had helped us bring into the world. We thanked him for taking such good care of us and I jokingly reminded him that I would not be into work the next day.

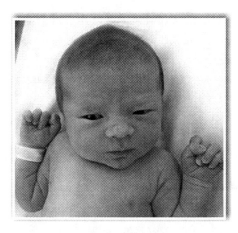

When Jeff brought Nicholas to me, tears welled up in my eyes. I was amazed that such tiny hands and feet could have kicked and punched so hard. He weighed in at 7 pounds, 1 ounce, and was 19.5 inches long. He really was a little peanut and he was all ours.

Jeff had called my parents when we learned I was completely dilated and the happy grandparents arrived a mere thirty minutes after Nicholas was born. My mom and dad kissed me on the forehead and then it was all Nicholas after that. My heart swelled to see my parents holding my son and cooing to him. I thought I would never get to experience such a moment, yet here it was right before me, and it was an incredible moment indeed. Nicholas started to cry so the nurse brought us a small bottle of formula. I was thrilled to feed my son for the very first time, and he ate like a champ. My breakfast soon arrived and I had my first nausea-free meal in a very long time. We moved to our postpartum room soon after that. My parents left to grab some breakfast and Jeff took Nicholas to have his first bath. I was instructed to get some sleep, but that was impossible. I was exhausted but lay in bed replaying the events of the past twenty-four hours.

Jeff soon returned with Nicholas, who was even cuter than before. The nurse had brushed his hair and cleaned him up and he was just precious. Even then I knew he had my hair and eyes, but he looked like Jeff with his nose and cheeks. I thought back to our transfer day and knew without a doubt that the embryologist had most definitely brought us the correct embies. A few short hours later, my sister and her son arrived to meet our little guy. From first touch, our sons bonded and my sister and I smiled to see her son gently watch over this newly arrived tiny bundle.

Jen's Mom Remembers

Regardless of what doctrine some religions might preach regarding IVF, follow your heart and do not listen to anybody else. I see it this way: if we humans were not supposed to unlock the miracle of conception and overcome medical impossibilities of creating new life, then we would not be given the brains to do so. Some say IVF is an evil thing to do. I dare them to tell me that after looking at my little grandson, so created and conceived, as he stands beautiful, bright, healthy and lovable, a human miracle and a creation of God.

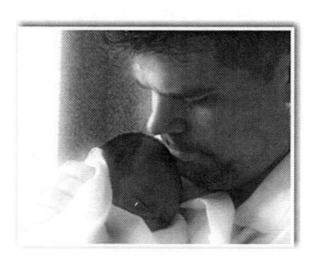

Later that night, Jeff, Nicholas and I snuggled in bed and enjoyed quiet time together as a new family. There had been so many dark, sad days in our life, but those were all behind us now. We had a permanent ray of sunshine in our hearts and souls to carry us through anything that lay ahead. On July 20, 2001, Jeff and I became infertility survivors, all thanks to modern medicine, caring physicians, and our resolve and determination as a couple to risk everything for the chance at becoming parents. We had asked God to bring us a child. In his wisdom he sent us Nicholas to mend our broken hearts, to join our souls forever, and to remind us each day where we had been and where we were going.

PART TWO

The Baby Chase

Chapter Four

Life as an Infertile Couple

The Good, the Bad, and the Ugly

According to the Centers for Disease Control (CDC), in 2002 about 1.2 million women of reproductive age in the United States had an infertility-related medical appointment within the previous twelve months, and 10 percent had an infertility-related medical visit at some point in the past.[1] The National Survey of Family Growth reports 7.4 percent of married women, or about 2.1 million women, were infertile in 2002.[2] According to the CDC's 2003 Assisted Reproductive Technologies (ART) Report, the most recent data available at the time of this book's printing, the number of assisted reproductive technology cycles performed in the United States has almost doubled, from 64,681 cycles in 1996 to 122,872 in 2003.[3] The number of couples affected by infertility is astounding. The data truly shows that infertile couples are not struggling alone.

Not all infertility couples will utilize in vitro fertilization to achieve pregnancy. Some will find success with Clomid or intrauterine insemination. Some will choose to adopt. Many will never seek assistance and remain childless. Regardless what path these couples travel, all infertility couples share in their struggles, their heartaches and their altered views of the "naturally" conceiving population. Infertility transcends all income brackets, all nationalities and all age groups. There is no typical appearance to an infertile couple. We are your coworkers, your neighbors and your friends.

Of those affected by infertility, it is likely that only a small portion of us will share our conception difficulties with anyone other than our physician. Infertility is a condition of inadequacy. There are often feelings of shame, guilt and anger toward ourselves and those around us. Sadly, so many of us never find a support network and don't realize all of these issues are common ones. Although it is important to understand the mechanisms and treatments of infertility, it is equally important that we openly face our feelings of being unable to conceive without the aid of medical intervention.

What most infertile women don't realize is that we have all dealt with the terrible swing of emotions when faced with someone else's pregnancy. Anyone struggling to overcome their infertility has a love of children. We would never endure all that we do or dedicate so much of our lives to achieving pregnancy ourselves if it wasn't for that strong love and enjoyment of little ones. It is always a blessing when a child is born. Their sweet innocence reminds us all of the good in the world and of the possibilities held by the future. The pudgy-cheeked smile of a baby can make any day seem bright. But often the intense joy we feel is replaced with sadness for that which we cannot achieve ourselves.

The ache of an infertile woman's heart is deep and all consuming. Some days it is hard to think of anything but our empty arms. It is not that we are self-centered and can think only of ourselves, but rather it is that we don't have a way of coping with the weight we feel is crushing our spirit. Our world is filled with pregnancy and babies through commercials, songs, conversations and interactions. We come face to face with our inadequacies everyday, whether we want to or not. Avoidance is simply impossible for those of us battling infertility.

That leaves us with very few options for coping. Many of us slip into depression when we feel overwhelmed by the obstacles in front of us. It is disheartening to face a negative pregnancy test, again and again. It is difficult to explain to our husband or loved one why we feel so blue. We don't want to hear that we are young and have plenty of time. We don't want to be told that we are trying too hard and should just relax. We only want the pain to stop, for this incredible longing to disappear. It is difficult to look forward to the future when it appears so dark over the horizon. Until we come to understand our diagnosis or undergo fertility treatments, there is no light to guide us. We often feel alone and lost in a cold and barren land. Our infertility is the black cloud that follows us through life, reminding us over and over again that we may never be a mother, a father or a grandparent. For the majority of us, our diagnosis of infertility is a lifelong diagnosis. Although blocked tubes may re-open, or a man with a low sperm count may one day father a child, the occurrence of this is not enough to hang our hopes on. The realization is, we may very well never experience the joy of conceiving a child, and that is a difficult thought to deal with on a daily basis.

For many of us, our sadness is compounded by intense feelings of guilt. In situations where it is purely a female factor or purely a male factor, the affected person must carry the burden of a childless home. Whether we have spoken the words or only thought them, the idea that our partner would be better off with someone else is a common one. "If you married someone else you could have children," or "If it wasn't for me, you could have children." For all the pain we carry inside for being responsible for our inability to conceive, we also carry the guilt of hurting our partner. Of course, it is not something we do intentionally and, most often, our loved one would never lay full blame at our feet, but we own their pain as much as we own ours. Guilt can be quite the demon. Oftentimes guilt makes us lash out at the ones we love because we are so hard on ourselves. We take every comment as an attack or a judgment. If we constantly point the finger at ourselves, then our partners must be pointing at us as well. How could they possibly see past what is so glaringly obvious: *The sound of a child's laugh may never echo through this house because of me. I hate myself for that.*

And with the self-hate comes anger at the world around us. *Why is it that so many unwanted babies are born when I desperately want one but am denied? Why will the government spend thousands and thousands of dollars to care for those same unwanted children but won't provide me with the opportunity to become a self-supporting parent? Why does my cash flow, my credit rating, or my insurance company get to decide if I am worthy of parenthood?* So many questions, yet never any good answers.

We begin to loathe a society that places such emphasis on conceiving, as if we are less a person if we never procreate. Yes, I want to have a child, but does everyone need to make me feel selfish or inadequate if I haven't achieved that goal by age 25 or 30, or even 40? We feel like punching the next person who says, "You don't understand, you're not a parent." We want to scream back, "No, you don't understand!" Others' insensitivity can hit us like a truck, often leaving us dazed wondering if they really just said that. Other insensitive comments include wonderful things such as, "God chooses who should and shouldn't have children," or "You don't want kids, your hips will get big," or even, "Get a dog instead, they are more obedient." Of course, there are always the seemingly endless comments of "When are you going to have kids? You better hurry up before time runs out and you're spoiled with no responsibilities except for yourselves." To be pummeled by friends and family for not maintaining the status quo, all the while dealing with terrible self-hatred and self-pity, seems like rather cruel punishment.

Do we feel sorry for ourselves? Oh yes, we do. We feel as though we are being punished unjustly. We follow the rules. We pay our taxes. We lead a good life. We expect to have the same opportunity as everyone else when it comes to getting pregnant, but instead we seem to get the short end of the stick, time and time again. But for all our self-pity, the absolute last thing we want from anyone else is pity. Far and above this, we desire understanding. Understanding for the pain we endure, understanding for the way this diagnosis affects every aspect of our lives, and understanding for our inability to give up on our dream, no matter the cost of chasing it.

All of these emotions lie just beneath the surface. Some days we wage a war against ourselves to not be angry today, to not cry today, to not think about having a child for one lousy day, leaving us exhausted and beaten down. Other days, we see hope and possibility in the pregnant woman next to us, the small child tugging at mommy's hand, and, we think, *my time will come. I have faith.*

Given such complex emotions, is it any wonder so many of us come to the breaking point in our marriage? Each partner must battle his or her own demons and face their partner's as well. With so many intense emotions, the strain can tug at even the strongest ties. Those of us who recognize the negative impact these emotions have on our relationship often step back, re-evaluate our lives, and make changes to ensure we maintain that special relationship with our loved one. Whether we take a break from trying to conceive, seek counseling to deal with the stress of infertility, opt to no longer cycle or decide to live childless, we take back control and regain emotional stability. Unfortunately, many of us spiral down and become buried under the weight of what faces us each day and slowly wedge a wall between ourselves and our loved one.

The lesson learned here is that any or all of these emotions are completely normal. It doesn't make anyone a bad person to feel hate, self-pity, or guilt. It's okay to have days of sadness, to cry at commercials or to bubble over with joy when holding a baby. Dealing with infertility can take much from us, but it can also give us what we may not have had before. Infertility forces us to educate ourselves about our bodies, about the diagnosis we have been given and about the different treatment options available to us. It drives us to become stronger and more determined in all aspects of our life, whether it is getting our bodies in better physical shape or setting goals for our jobs and finances. Our infertility demands that we work harder in order to reach our goal of parenthood. We must look ourselves in the eye and move past all the negativity in order to put our demons in their place.

We may face our infertility every day, but we don't have to let it rule our lives. We can ride out every bump and pothole on the path. We can survive the bad days and enjoy the good days. And we can allow ourselves to be more than women trying to conceive. We can be lovers, daughters, sisters, friends. It is one of the most difficult things we will ever do, to rise above the heartache and hardships, to move forward when it is easier to stand still, to take control in a situation beyond our control. But we all have the strength within to carry us through the difficult days of trying to conceive. Whether our journey takes us beyond our diagnosis or not, we must all find peace within our hearts and souls for the path we have been chosen to travel.

Chapter Five

The Phases of an IVF Cycle

Understanding a Complex Undertaking

An in vitro fertilization cycle can seem overwhelming on first encounter, but becomes very manageable and understandable when broken down into phases. As an IVFer, you probably wish to actively participate in your healthcare and your journey to parenthood. This requires a certain amount of commitment, because it isn't enough just to learn the stages of a cycle and blindly go through them. Rather, it is important to fully understand the specific goals of each phase so that, first and foremost, you have realistic expectations and second, that you make positive contributions. This may be dosing your medications accurately and administering them consistently, following up appropriately with your clinic, or communicating effectively with your physician. Make yourself aware of the ultimate goals for each phase and focus your energy into achieving them. Timing your medications correctly and not missing an appointment are much more manageable goals than becoming pregnant. Set your sights on the end of each stage— a very reasonable timeframe to work towards when facing the seemingly endless weeks of an IVF cycle. Take time to truly understand the path you are about to travel and step with confidence along the road to parenthood.

Although not every couple will pass through each phase of an in vitro fertilization cycle, and not every couple will devote the same amount of time to each phase, the following chapters outline each in detail to make it easier to understand the process in general. The phases of an in vitro fertilization cycle include the preparation phase; the suppression phase (not all couples will undergo suppression); the stimulation phase (the hCG trigger shot is given at the end of the stimulation phase); the egg retrieval phase; the embryo transfer phase; the two week wait (this is a general term as the time between embryo transfer and the beta blood test varies); and the weeks beyond the beta. Typically, you will not see reference to the weeks beyond the beta as part of an in vitro cycle, but I believe these weeks are intimately tied to a cycle and should be included for closure.

Chapter Six

Preparing to Cycle

*preparation...suppression...stimulation...egg retrieval...
embryo transfer...two week wait...and beyond*

Ready...Set...Wait?

Choosing a Reproductive Endocrinologist

When you make the decision to pursue in vitro fertilization, your first step in preparing to cycle is choosing a reproductive endocrinologist. Even in instances where you must remain in-network for insurance coverage purposes, there are always choices regarding who will manage your cycle. It is important to do some research on each reproductive endocrinologist (RE) and clinic to find someone who best suits your needs. If you do not have insurance coverage and therefore do not have any restrictions as to whom you trust your care to, you need not limit your selection to local clinics. Many fertility clinics will work with you even if you live out-of-state, only requiring you to travel to the clinic once you reach the stimulation phase of a cycle where close monitoring is essential.

Reproductive Endocrinologist

A subspecialist in obstetrics and gynecology who deals with reproductive endocrinology and infertility-related issues in women, and who has successfully completed a graduate education program at least thirty-six months in duration.

So how do you begin to narrow the choices to just a few doctors whom you'd like to contact regarding your fertility care? This will be a very personal decision, as you will have your own opinion about what is most important. Factors to consider might include the doctor's bedside manner and personality; success rates; location; availability; cost; and procedures offered. You may prefer to find a doctor with the highest success rate, wishing to give yourself the best statistical chance of success. You might choose a program based on cost in order to avoid over-stretching your finances or you might search for a physician with a caring reputation with her patients, making your experience more personal. You may need to find a physician with specialized surgical techniques or with adequate experience dealing with your specific diagnosis.

Write down what criteria you'd like your physician to meet in order of importance and formulate a list of your top three or four choices. Individual clinic Web sites will help you narrow your selection based on location, procedures offered and cost. The CDC Web site (http://www.cdc.gov/reproductivehealth/ART/index.htm) provides success rates for clinics nationwide as well as statistics pertaining to age, diagnosis and other information. Online message boards may also be a source for patient recommendations as well as criticisms. Following your research, take the time to contact your first and second choices and ask for a consultation appointment. If your physician of choice is not local, many will provide phone consultations so as to negate the need for you to travel initially.

Reasons You May Be Declined as a Patient

Yes, there is the possibility that you will not be accepted as a patient at a fertility clinic. This may be due to substance abuse, advanced maternal age, a high Day 3 FSH level, indications of physical abuse, severe marital discord or coercion of one partner by another. Use of illicit drugs or alcohol abuse will raise a red flag and hinder your chances of acceptance at a clinic. Your age will also be a determining factor. Many clinics have a maximum maternal age they will accept because the chances of a successful cycle decline significantly with increasing maternal age. The cut-off age will vary from clinic to clinic, but typically no RE will accept a woman older than fifty into his IVF program. In recent years the world has been stunned by headlines reporting babies being born to women of significantly advanced age (in terms of reproductive age) following an IVF cycle. It is important to realize that often times these women falsify information, claiming to be much younger than they really are, which in turn allows them to be accepted into an in vitro fertilization program. A high Day 3 FSH indicates inadequate ovarian function and is a red flag for poor cycle outcome. Again, each clinic will have specific guidelines regarding what qualifies as too high of an FSH level. Should your RE suspect there is physical abuse in your relationship, she may decline you as a patient. This is also true in cases where one partner is attempting to force the other partner into doing an IVF cycle against their will. Refusal to accept you as a patient for reasons of physical abuse or coercion is supported by the Hippocratic Oath.

The Embryologist

You need to consider the qualifications of your reproductive endocrinologist, but it may also be prudent to weigh the qualifications of the embryologist your RE works with when choosing a program for your in vitro cycle. With assisted reproductive technology, clinical embryologists are responsible for preparing the egg and sperm samples, providing the proper conditions for fertilization, and maintaining the necessary conditions for growth to occur.

Embryologist

Your embryologist will at minimum have a Bachelor Degree in embryology, biology, microbiology, genetics or biochemistry.

The embryologist performs intracytoplasmic sperm injection (ICSI) and assisted hatching (AZH/AH) to aid in fertilization and implantation respectively. Both are very delicate and precise techniques requiring an experienced and skilled hand. Clinical embryologists are also responsible for facilitating the growth and preservation of the developing embryo. They are the ones who will watch over your embies and monitor their progress. If you choose to freeze your embryos, it is the embryologist who will perform the cryopreservation. Different embryologists and labs may have different success rates. This may be more of a consideration for you if you have cycled previously without success, but it bears mentioning to emphasize the numerous factors involved when it comes to having a successful in vitro fertilization cycle.

"For I dipt into the future, far as human eye could see, saw the vision of the world, and all the wonder that would be."—*Lord Alfred Tennyson*

Managing IVF Costs

When dealing with insurance companies, always doublecheck that your RE is covered under your plan provisions and always have your clinic call to obtain specific coverage for in vitro fertilization procedures. Many plans might state there is no coverage but the testing and monitoring of a cycle as well as medications may be covered with a co-pay. Most clinics now have a person who specifically deals with insurance companies and coverage plans to help you get the maximum benefits to which you are entitled. Sometimes terminology for procedures makes the difference between coverage and no coverage, so allow the clinic to help you when dealing with your insurance company. Should your insurance refuse coverage, contact your local state representative to determine if your state mandates fertility treatment coverage. Living in a state which mandates coverage does not guarantee you coverage, as there are specific criteria companies must meet to be bound by this mandate. Take the time to investigate all avenues before embarking on this long and stressful journey to make it the least expensive and most productive experience for you.

If you are unlucky enough to have very limited coverage or no coverage, now is the time to prepare yourself for the enormous financial strain of an IVF cycle. Many clinics now offer financing options and there are lenders offering loans specifically for fertility treatments as well as employer plans constructed to help with medical costs. Some couples will take out home equity loans while others will pay for treatments with their credit cards. Only you can decide how far you are willing or able to stretch in order to cycle. Sit down together and scour your finances for ways to save here and there—even small cutbacks can add up in the long run. Ask family and friends to give money rather than gifts for birthdays and holidays—and thank them for contributing to your baby fund.

Other options include free or low-cost IVF cycles offered through various clinics as part of a clinical trial. Visit the CDC Web site (http://www.clinicaltrials.org) for a listing of current trials specifically for fertility treatment. These clinical trials often offer free medications or cycles at reduced cost in exchange for your participation. Bear in mind, most trials will have very strict guidelines for participation and you may have to search to find one you qualify for or wait several months to actually begin a clinical trial.

Some clinics offer shared-risk programs where you pay for multiple cycles in advance to receive a discounted rate. Should you not achieve pregnancy, part of your money is refundable. Read these agreements carefully to make sure you understand what qualifies as a cycle and how much of your payment will be refunded should your cycle be unsuccessful. If your cycle is canceled, does it count as one of your shared-risk cycles? Does a frozen embryo transfer (FET) count as a shared-risk cycle or do only fresh cycles (cycles in which eggs are retrieved and fertilized thus producing embryos) count?

It is also possible to participate as an egg donor in order to cover the cost of your own cycle. Again, there are strict guidelines which set age limitations and specify the timeline of your egg donation and IVF cycle. Always make sure you enter these agreements with open eyes and realistic expectations. Finally, consider asking your clinic for donated medications. This is the one time it is okay to accept used medications, as your clinic will have guidelines in place to ensure the medications you receive are safe and the proper dosage for your cycle.

"Courage is not the absence of fear, but rather the judgment that something else is more important than fear."—*Ambrose Redmoon*

How Men and Women React to Cycling

Another aspect of the preparation phase is preparing emotionally for what lies ahead. In vitro fertilization is likely to be one of the most emotionally draining undertakings of your life. Understanding how men and women react to and cope with the stresses of cycling differently may ease some of the emotional turmoil during your cycle. You may already have a strained relationship due to your struggle with infertility. Months or years of trying to conceive can take their toll on any relationship and open communication will help you and your partner come closer together rather than drift further apart.

HINT for COUPLES

Before embarking on your IVF journey, agree to share the responsibilities of your cycle so that you both feel equally committed. Prepare and administer injections together, be present together for ultrasounds whenever possible, and promise to always be honest about how you are feeling. An IVF cycle should ALWAYS be a team effort.

—————————————————

In terms of cycling, women experience greater emotional distress concerning their diagnosis and treatment compared to men. Men will often prefer not to discuss all the aspects of cycling. They take the approach of problem solving. "Tell me what I need to do and when, and I will do my part." They keep their emotions in check for most of the cycle and usually do not share their experiences or concerns with anyone, including their loved one. Lack of expression by the man does not indicate a disinterested or unemotional partner; it is simply his coping mechanism. Women are quite different. Women tend to express all the incredible emotions tugging at them as they cycle, be it sadness, concern or anger. The "what if" scenario plays over and over in their minds and fear of bad consequences for not following instructions to the letter often lingers in the back of their minds. It is important to remember that an IVF cycle experience for women is quite different than for men because women are subjected to more invasive procedures and the manipulation of their hormones. Many of the emotions women must deal with are directly influenced by the medications they are being injected with and therefore these emotions are somewhat beyond their control. With men and women experiencing such different emotions, it is easy to see how a wall can quickly build between two otherwise very loving individuals. Your partner should always be your strongest support, but if he is unable to express himself at the same level as you, then by all means try to understand that and seek support from others.

Although you may feel uncomfortable doing so, joining a support group can have a dramatic, positive impact on your cycle and your relationship with your loved one. In vitro fertilization is extremely stressful, entails many ups and downs, and steals control from you. If you combine all of that and find your partner is unable or unwilling to talk through all these emotions, it is easy to find yourself feeling abandoned and lost. No one should feel they must tackle this alone. A support group provides a forum for sharing all the ugliness, sadness and happiness that encircles the diagnosis of infertility and in vitro. Venting about the little things that upset you can keep emotions from building to the boiling point and often, when you find yourself feeling very low, a support group can remind you of the good lying just beneath the surface. Fellow IVFers understand the complex emotions that ravage a couple during a cycle and can offer comfort and stability when stress levels reach their peak. The common ground of a good support group will give you a stable foundation to hold you up and give you strength during your cycle and beyond.

HINT for WOMEN

Find an online support group that offers cycle buddies. Cycle buddies are members going through an IVF cycle at the same time and provide a wonderful outlet for sharing all the daily ups and downs while giving a point of reference to what others experience with each phase.

Choosing an Online Support Group

So, how do you choose a good online support group? Above all else, do not take this decision lightly. Unless you plan to be a "lurker"—someone who regularly visits a group without ever actually posting messages or joining discussions—you will be sharing a very personal experience with others. In a public group, meaning one that anyone on the Internet can view, your messages may be seen by hundreds, or even thousands, of people, not all of whom will be struggling with infertility. Chances are, at some point you will vent, you will cry, and you will seek advice. It is important to find a group that fits you and gives you the support you need and deserve. More and more personal support groups are popping up on the Internet and most infertility organizations and infertility-related companies now offer support groups. Take your time searching for and sifting through all the available choices. Remember, not all support groups are of the same caliber. Unfortunately, many personal support groups provide more opinion than medical fact and are often subject to personal disputes and lack of supervision. Personal groups are more likely to become inactive or be closed due to member discord or loss of interest by management. On the positive side, personal support groups can be filled with very knowledgeable members with vast combined personal experience.

Larger professional support groups often have medical staff willing to answer questions and are less likely to suddenly close. However, these support groups are more likely to require membership fees, often have targeted advertising and may impose strict member guidelines that can interrupt the flow of discussions. Any group can fall victim to ill-meaning individuals who feed off the emotional instability of cycling couples. Safety should always be a high priority when participating in an online support group.

The following guidelines can help ensure that your experience with a support group is a positive one:

- Consider using an anonymous screen name or only use your first name when posting. This gives you privacy from any disingenuous lurkers as well as any clinic staff or coworkers who may check message boards.

- Use an anonymous e-mail account (such as Hotmail or Yahoo!), or set up a secondary e-mail account with your ISP.

- NEVER post your e-mail address or personal information in a public group and use caution in private groups. Spiders crawl the web searching for e-mail addresses to add to spam lists and again, you cannot account for everyone who might be reading your posts. If you must post your e-mail, write it out with spaces or write it in sentence form so that spiders cannot pick it up as they crawl the web (i.e., IVFer at mail accounts dot com).

- Never disregard the instructions of your RE based on comments made in a group. Your doctor has all the information of your case and is a trained specialist. Misinformation abounds on the Internet and posted information should always be taken with a grain of salt. If you have concerns, by all means contact your physician and discuss these concerns with her.

- Steer clear of support groups with high membership numbers but few posted messages. This could be a clue about a poor group where members simply leave or indicates there are many lurkers who are unwilling or unable to provide support. Find a group where you know you will have meaningful interactions.

- Always follow your gut instincts. If you feel uncomfortable in a group, move on and find a new group. Again, many groups will fall victim to malicious members only looking to cause trouble and some will be unfortunate enough to have members there for purposes other than support, going so far as to fabricate stories to gain the trust and sympathy of fellow group members.

- Join more than one group. This allows you to test drive a support group and find a place to call home. Never share information from one group with another; respect for each group's privacy should be a given.

- Join a support group specifically for IVF/FET or find a group that includes message boards specifically for IVF/FET. The stress and potential complications of an in vitro cycle are much different than those of Clomid cycles or intrauterine insemination (IUI) cycles.

- NEVER buy used medications offered in a group. Any reputable support group will forbid the selling or trading of used medications. It is extremely unsafe to buy used medications online because there is no way of ensuring these medications were stored properly or verifying the medications are as labeled.

- Be honest and open in your messages and caring for others' feelings. Share your experiences so that others can benefit and so that you can find others who have "been there done that." Reaffirmation that what you are feeling and going through is completely normal can be a lifesaver during an IVF cycle.

Lifestyle Changes

Whether your preparation phase begins weeks or months prior to your cycle, now is the time to make lifestyle changes that will improve your chances of achieving pregnancy. This means lowering your caffeine intake, avoiding alcohol and saying goodbye to cigarettes/nicotine. Get yourself in the mindset of no longer using ibuprofen, as you must avoid this while cycling. Your RE will either give you samples or a prescription for prenatal vitamins to begin prior to your cycle. Adequate folic acid intake is essential during pregnancy to prevent neural tube defects in your baby, as is adequate iron stores to avoid anemia in pregnancy. Think of these lifestyle changes as wonderful markers for the months of pregnancy that may be just over the horizon.

Also prepare yourself for a likely decline in your sex life as you progress through your IVF cycle. Not only does the stress affect your intimacy, but the physical changes your body undergoes can actually make sexual intercourse uncomfortable or even painful. It is important that you both realize that a decrease in sexual activity is a very real possibility and that it in no way signals a loss of love or need for intimacy between you. In fact, the need for intimacy increases during a cycle with sensual touching, hugging and kissing often being the moments that keep an otherwise very clinical undertaking very personal and passionate. Try to surround yourself with positive energy when preparing to cycle, as pre-cycle depression can negatively impact IVF cycle outcomes.[4] Educate yourselves about the changes about to happen in all aspects of your lives and face them together as a couple so that when all is said and done, you still have the same amazing relationship and love for each other that brought you to the doorstep of your RE.

Potential Complications of Cycling

Prior to beginning your IVF cycle, you will also participate in patient education programs regarding proper injection techniques. Numerous consent forms will need to be completed regarding potential side effects, risks and complications, type of embryo transfer, number of embryos to be transferred, cryopreservation, and becoming a donor. Please realize that although serious complications do not occur frequently, the potential complications of IVF can be life threatening.

POTENTIAL COMPLICATIONS

- Ovarian hyperstimulation syndrome (OHSS)
- Ectopic pregnancy
- Multiple gestation (twins, triplets, etc.)
- Infection (caused by injections or egg retrieval procedure)
- Ovarian torsion

If you have any questions, do not understand any part of the procedure, or are concerned about potential complications, now is the time to ask your physician for clarification. Don't be afraid, don't feel stupid and don't be intimidated. Be informed! Realistic expectations are essential and a sound understanding of what lies ahead crucial. As a well-informed patient, you will be able to contribute to your healthcare more effectively and improve your chances of success.

Updating Your Will

You and your partner should update your will. It is important to make a legal statement regarding the fate of your embryos in the event something happens to one or both of you. This statement should cover several scenarios. If you both become physically or mentally incapacitated, or if you both die, do you wish to give someone the right to determine the fate of your embryos? Do you wish to have your embryos donated for research or ethically destroyed? What if only one of you becomes incapacitated or passes? Would you like your surviving partner to have the right to do as he or she wishes with the embryos, even if that means possibly using the embryos to achieve pregnancy with another person? These are important decisions to make and should not be made lightly. Discuss your feelings openly and take the time to update your will to ensure your wishes are carried out. If you do not have a will, get one. Your embryos are too precious to leave their fate to emotionally-strained loved ones or, worse, the courts.

Time Management

Now is the time to manage your work schedule to allow for blood work, ultrasounds, egg retrieval, and embryo transfer. IVF is a closely monitored and precisely timed process. Make sure to plan your life accordingly to avoid conflicts before they can even occur.

HINT for COUPLES

Determine in advance what vacation days, sick days or personal days you have available at work to give you the time off you'll need for your IVF cycle.

When you enter the stimulation phase, blood draws are done more frequently, as are ultrasounds, to monitor the growth of your follicles. If you have a physically strenuous job, your workload and schedule may need to be adjusted during the stimulation phase due to your enlarging ovaries so as to lessen the chances of ovarian torsion (a condition where the ovary twists on itself, cutting off the blood supply). Plan to take off the day of your egg retrieval. Some women experience only mild soreness while others may be quite sore or feel ill from the medications used during the procedure. The hCG trigger shot and the transfer of embryos are two of the most precisely timed aspects of a cycle and it is imperative that your schedule allows you to be on time for both your trigger shot and your transfer.

Possible Pre-Cycle Testing and Procedures

The testing aspect of the preparation phase has the widest variation among couples as each couple's medical history and diagnosis determine what is required during the preparation phase. You may already know your diagnosis and may not need to have as much testing performed as another couple.

Possible Testing and Procedures

- Hepatitis
- HIV
- Pap smear
- Cultures
- CBC
- Thyroid levels
- Immune testing
- Day 3 FSH
- Antral follicle count
- Ovarian volume
- Hysterosonogram

- Hysteroscopy
- Hysterosalpingogram
- Exploratory laparoscopy
- Mock transfer
- Semen analysis
- Sperm extraction procedures

You and your partner will be tested for hepatitis and HIV. If one was not recently performed by your referring physician, your RE may perform a Pap smear and pelvic examination (with or without cultures) as well as general blood work such as a complete blood count and thyroid levels. If indicated, you may also undergo immune testing.

Ovarian Reserve Assessment

Ovarian reserve testing allows your reproductive endocrinologist to assess your functional ovarian age and indicates your reproductive potential. The ovarian reserve assessment predicts how your ovaries will respond to stimulation medications and what your chances are for achieving success with your in vitro fertilization cycle. Decreased ovarian reserve (DOR) is a strong predictor of poor cycle outcome and may either prevent you from cycling or impact the protocol your doctor chooses. The three tests your RE may perform to assess your ovarian reserve include: Day 3 FSH, antral follicle count, and ovarian volume.

Day 3 FSH

Many clinics will require a Day 3 FSH and estradiol level to check for ovarian reserve. The Day 3 FSH test is a blood test done typically on the third day of your menstrual cycle, although it may be done on Day 2 or Day 4, and measures the level of follicle-stimulating hormone. As you age, your ovaries become less responsive to hormonal influences and your body increases FSH in an attempt to force your ovaries to produce follicles and eggs. An elevated Day 3 FSH level is associated with a poor response to stimulation medications during an IVF cycle and lower pregnancy rates (likely due to a decline in egg quality).[5] Follicle-stimulating hormone normally fluctuates from day to day and from menstrual cycle to menstrual cycle, so your RE may perform this test more than once should your level come back elevated. Your physician will likely check the estradiol level at the same time she checks the FSH level. An elevated estradiol level may indicate an aging ovary or the presence of follicular cysts remaining from the previous menstrual cycle.

Antral Follicle Count

Antral follicles are those follicles present at the beginning of the menstrual cycle that are awaiting stimulation by gonadotropins. To determine your total antral follicle count, your RE will perform a transvaginal ultrasound to count the sum of follicles in the right ovary and the left ovary, if both are present. The total antral follicle count decreases with age.[6] Your RE may asses your antral follicle count as it predicts ovarian responsiveness to stimulation medications during an in vitro fertilization cycle.[7] Typically, the higher the antral follicle count the better the response to stimulation medications.[8] If you are older than thirty-five, however, your response to stimulation medications and your chances of achieving pregnancy are likely to be diminished regardless of your antral count.[9] One theory suggests that ovaries with a low antral follicle count are incapable of significantly increasing blood flow to developing follicles, which may lead to poorer embryo quality. An antral follicle count of less than five indicates decreased ovarian reserve and is often associated with a significantly decreased pregnancy rate.[10]

Ovarian Volume

The ovarian volume assessment is another way for your RE to evaluate your ovarian reserve, as the two are correlated. Small ovaries (those with a diminished volume) have a poor response to gonadotropin stimulation and are associated with a high cancellation rate during IVF.[11]

Hysteroscopy/Hysterosonogram/Hysterosalpingogram

You may also be required to have one or more of the following procedures performed: hysteroscopy, hysterosonogram and/or hysterosalpingogram. The hysteroscopy and hysterosonogram procedures are diagnostic tools that allow your physician to evaluate the uterine structure. The hysteroscopy procedure provides your physician with a direct view of the inside of your uterus through a small scope, which is inserted through the cervix. The hysterosonogram uses ultrasound and fluid to delineate the inner surface of your uterus. Abnormalities such as fibroids, polyps and uterine septums are visible during these procedures and speak to the ability of your uterus to carry a pregnancy to term. The hysterosalpingogram involves injecting dye into the uterine cavity and monitoring for spillage of dye from the Fallopian tubes. This allows your RE to evaluate the inner surfaces of your uterus as well as the patency of your tubes (to check if your tubes are open or blocked). Blocked tubes will not allow dye to spill and partially blocked tubes will significantly decrease dye spillage. It is important to realize that if you have blocked tubes you may experience significant pain following an HSG. Any dye that remains in the uterus or that spills into the pelvic cavity will be absorbed by your body.

Exploratory Laparoscopy

Depending on your medical history, your doctor may decide to perform an exploratory laparoscopy to look for endometriosis, adhesions, tubal disease, and other disease entities or conditions. If pre-cycle testing reveals a uterine fibroid or septum, you will need to have these surgically removed prior to the start of your cycle.

Mock Transfer

Some, but not all, clinics will perform what is called a mock transfer. Some perform this during the preparation phase while others perform it in the midst of the actual IVF cycle. A small catheter is inserted into the uterus to measure the depth required for optimal embryo placement. As each woman's uterus is different, this gives your RE a snapshot of your uterus and alerts her to any difficulties that might be encountered, such as a severely tilted uterus or a stenotic (narrowed) cervix. Should your mock transfer suggest embryo placement will be difficult, your cycle may be switched to a zygote intrafallopian transfer (ZIFT) procedure, where the zygotes (fertilized eggs) are surgically placed in the Fallopian tube rather than in the uterus. If the mock transfer reveals your cervix to be very narrow, your physician will likely address this prior to your transfer with medical intervention that will open the cervix to allow easy passage of the catheter.

Although you must endure the majority of testing, your partner will be tested for hepatitis and HIV, as previously mentioned, and will need a semen analysis. Depending on the semen analysis results, your partner may also need to undergo a sperm extraction procedure.

Semen Analysis

The semen analysis looks for concentration, morphology and motility of sperm. In other words, the analysis evaluates the number of sperm, how they look, and how they move. In general, a normal semen analysis reports:

- Volume of 2.0 ml or greater
- pH of 7.2-8
- Concentration of 20 million/ml or greater
- Total count of 40 million/ejaculate or greater
- Motility of 50 percent or more with forward progression, or 25 percent or more with rapid movement within sixty minutes of ejaculation
- Vitality of 75 percent or greater and with fewer than one million white blood cells
- Morphology of 30 percent or more with normal forms

Concentrations less than 20 million/ml are considered sub-fertile but do not constitute infertility. Concentrations less than 5 million/ml are considered infertile. This means men with concentrations less than 20 million may take longer to impregnate their partners, but they are able to achieve pregnancy together. When the concentration drops below 5 million, conception is not likely to occur without assistance.[12]

Typically, sperm have an oval-shaped head with a single tail. Although fertile men will have a certain percentage of sperm with variations in shape, sperm with significant defects are not likely to or are unable to penetrate the egg. Motility (movement) is categorized as rapid progressive motility; slow or sluggish progressive motility; non-progressive motility; or no motility. Again, 50 percent or more of the sperm should show forward progression or 25 percent or more should show rapid forward progression.[13]

Reference to agglutination may also appear in the semen analysis report. Agglutination is a condition where motile sperm stick to each other and is suggestive of immunologic factor infertility. It is important to remember that there is variability in a semen sample among the population and with an individual. To diagnose a man with consistently abnormal sperm production, more than a single specimen is required. Should your partner have a normal semen analysis the egg and sperm will likely be placed together with unassisted fertilization. In the event your partner has an abnormal semen analysis, the embryologist will assist fertilization with injection of the sperm into the egg, also known as intracytoplasmic sperm injection (ICSI). With severe male factor involving limited concentration, your partner may undergo a surgical technique to extract the sperm. With surgical sperm extraction, the sperm are prepared and frozen, and later thawed for use at the time of egg retrieval.

HINT for GUYS

Discreetly bring along a magazine that "peaks" your interest for the semen analysis. This way, if your clinic doesn't have much of a selection, you are still able to produce a sample in the time allotted; this holds true for the semen analysis and the day of egg retrieval.

Sperm Extraction Procedures

If your diagnosis is severe male factor (infertility due to abnormalities with the man's sperm) your partner may undergo a sperm extraction procedure during the preparation phase. Examples of sperm extraction techniques include microepididymal sperm aspiration (MESA), percutaneous epididymal sperm aspiration (PESA) and testicular sperm aspiration (TESA). These specialized techniques allow extraction of sperm in cases where a typical semen sample would not yield enough quality sperm capable of fertilizing the retrieved eggs. Extracted sperm are frozen for use following the egg retrieval procedure.

Many of these tests (i.e. semen analysis, Pap smear, hepatitis, thyroid levels, and basic immune testing) will have been performed by your family doctor or gynecologist if they began an infertility work-up prior to referring you to a reproductive endocrinologist or if you previously attempted Clomid therapy or intrauterine insemination.

HINT for COUPLES

Gather your pertinent medical information prior to your consultation. Bring results from previous testing as well as any X-rays to avoid repetition and help lower costs.

Results of certain testing (i.e. CBC, hysterosonogram, hysteroscopy, hysterosalpingogram, immune testing, and Day 3 FSH) may alter the start date of your in vitro fertilization cycle. For example, if testing shows you to be severely anemic, you will need to start supplemental iron therapy to lessen your anemia prior to cycling. If your doctor finds a large fibroid, a large ovarian cyst, or a uterine septum, you may need to have it surgically removed before proceeding with your cycle. Although you are no doubt anxious to finally take steps toward your dream, your body needs to be as healthy as possible for the best outcome with your cycle. As with any endeavor, the preparation phase may well be the most time consuming, but it is essential to a successful outcome!

Tests with Expiration Dates

Remember, certain tests do have an expiration date. You may wait to attempt in vitro fertilization or take a long break between cycles (years in some instances). If you delay starting a cycle or are looking to cycle again several months down the line, tests such as the semen analysis and hysterosonogram will need to be repeated close to your cycle. This gives your clinic current information which helps determine if fertilization must be assisted as with intracytoplasmic sperm injection (ICSI) and allows them to reevaluate your uterus to confirm it is able to support a pregnancy. A Day 3 FSH and estradiol level may also be rechecked to assess your ovarian reserve—a strong marker for your ovaries' ability to produce eggs during the stimulation phase.

Overcoming Your Fear of Needles

During the preparation phase, you may find yourself facing your fear of needles and sharp objects, also called belonephobia or aichmophobia. If you have a fear of needles, the prospect of attempting in vitro fertilization can be terrifying. Needles are used throughout a cycle (blood draws, medication injections, egg retrieval and IVs), so there really is no way to avoid them.

HINT for COUPLES

Lay out all your medications, needles and supplies to make sure you are not missing anything. Check each vial for an expiration date and a secure seal. Take time to acquaint yourself with handling the needles and viewing them so they become more like everyday objects rather than objects of fear.

———————————

If you have a fear of needles, you must make a decision. Is your desire to conceive a child stronger than your fear of needles? If your desire for a baby is strong, you can and will find the strength to face your worries and fears. In order to overcome your fear, try to decipher why you dislike needles so much.

Do you fear the pain of a needle stick? If you are being suppressed, the needle used during this phase is very small, much smaller than the needle used to draw blood. Most women, even those afraid of needles, say they were pleasantly surprised when their first injection was completely painless and over so quickly. If you are not being suppressed, the needle used during the stimulation phase is larger, but again very tolerable and smaller than the needle used for blood draws. Remind yourself this is short-term pain and the payoff in the long-term is a child. Much as you tolerate waxing or plucking your bikini area or eyebrows, or endure having your ears pierced, you can survive the prick of a needle. Believe that you can. Know that you can.

Is your fear of needles due to a dislike of blood? During injections, you may occasionally have some slight leakage of blood, but a cotton ball or gauze pad can be placed over the blood quickly and be tossed without a second glance. There is always the chance your injection will inadvertently puncture a blood vessel, but the blood will be noticeable within the syringe upon pulling back and again, a quick gauze pad or Band-Aid over the area will block your view of the blood (remember, you never inject your medication if you see blood in the syringe when pulling back on the plunger). Again, you must take control and remind yourself that much like the blood of your menstrual cycle, this blood allows you to conceive a child. It will be the bringer of life to your small one for many months to come and will tie you to that same child forever.

Do you worry about infection? The risk of infection due to the injections of an in vitro cycle is very small as long as you follow antiseptic guidelines when preparing the area and syringe. It becomes second nature after the first few injections and is a simple routine to follow each time. Always wash your hands before touching the needles and syringes. Always inspect your medication and syringe for signs of contamination or damage. If a seal is broken, DO NOT use that item. If the tip of the needle is broken it should be safely discarded and NOT used. Never use a needle more than once. Always wipe the area well with an alcohol swab in either an outward spiraling circle from the center point or with a clean swipe across the area of injection. Don't go back and forth over the area in a scrubbing motion. If you've been outside or to the gym and the swab comes back dirty, it is always a safe bet to use another alcohol wipe to make sure the area is indeed clean. It is key to maintain your perspective when facing a fear of infection. Each day, your body faces an onslaught of potential sources of infection and wards them off through defense mechanisms. Take the same care you do in your day-to-day life and follow the same routine each time to help lessen the risks of infection.

Do you have sensitivity to the antiseptic smell? This can be overcome with aromatherapy. Fill your surroundings with the smell of fragrant candles or incense, or do your injections near an open window where the smell is much less noticeable. Try carrying a small sachet of fresh lavender to your blood draws to camouflage the sterile smell of the lab and relax your nerves. Consider brewing some fresh coffee at home to fill the air with wonderful aromas that will lift your spirit rather than instill apprehension.

First Injection Jitters

When you are ready to begin your first in vitro cycle, there can be an enormous amount of fear and anxiety that first injection night. It is a rather intense moment just to be finally starting a cycle and often those emotions can intensify apprehension about the first injection. It is very common to have shaking hands and feel a little sick to your stomach. So many times we refer to an IVF cycle as a roller coaster ride. That first injection night can often be as intense as the roller coaster's slow climb to the top before the first big drop. After talking about braving the roller coaster, you find yourself standing in line with the excitement building. As you make the slow climb upward, the tension builds further and further. A large part of that tension is due to your inability to see exactly what lies ahead. Take a deep breath, grab your loved one's hand and face that first drop head on. After that, everything will flow and you'll look back and think, "What was I so afraid of? It wasn't so bad after all." Remember, many couples before you have conquered their fear and you can too!

Overview of the Preparation Phase

- Find a reproductive endocrinologist you are comfortable with and who fits what you are looking for in a physician.
- Undergo testing to determine your cause of infertility and any contributing factors or potential stumbling blocks.
- Results from some testing may delay the start of your cycle.
- Prepare on all fronts—physically, emotionally, mentally and financially.
- Make arrangements at work to avoid scheduling conflicts before they can occur.
- Build a strong foundation to give yourself solid footing throughout your cycle.
- Join a support group or confide in a friend so you have support other than your partner for when the road gets really rough.
- Take a deep breath and always remember why you are taking on such a difficult challenge. No matter what lumps, bumps, dips or pitfalls you might find along the path, finally achieving pregnancy and having a child is worth it all…and then some!

Chapter Seven

The Suppression Phase

preparation...suppression...stimulation...egg retrieval...
embryo transfer...two week wait...and beyond

Cycling with a Blue Hue

The suppression phase is the down regulation portion of an IVF cycle. The main goal of this phase is to prevent the premature release of eggs before they can be retrieved by your reproductive endocrinologist (RE). Down regulation of the ovaries is achieved through the use of medications called gonadotropin-releasing hormone agonists (GnRHa).

Types of Suppression Medications

GENERIC NAME	TRADE NAME	HOW ADMINISTERED
Leuoprorelin	• Lupron • Enantone • Prostap	• SubQ • IM
Buserelin	• Suprafact • Supercur	• SubQ • IN
Nafarelin	Synarel	IN
Triptorelin	Decapeptyl	SubQ

SubQ—subcutaneous (just beneath the skin), IM—intramuscular (into the muscle), IN—intra-nasal (sniffed)

Subcutaneous injections are rapidly absorbed and remain at elevated concentrations for many hours. Since blood levels remain elevated for long periods, once-daily injections are adequate. The absorption from intra-nasal administration is unpredictable due to normal breakdown of the medication and some loss through swallowing medication that has dripped down the back of the throat. With this unpredictable absorption, a nasal spray is administered two to four times a day to ensure adequate blood concentrations.

REMEMBER

It is important to read the storage information for your medications as some need to be stored at specific temperatures. Improper storage may decrease the medication's potency and effectiveness.

Surviving the First Injection

Starting the suppression phase marks the beginning of an IVF cycle and the beginning of many needle sticks (unless, of course, your cycle does not include the suppression phase). Even those not afraid of needles will feel some apprehension as that first injection time approaches. Following are some suggestions to get you through that first injection and the many more to follow:

- Injections done closer to the belly button in an outward pattern are less painful. Injections done too high, too low or too far to either side will hurt more.
- Icing the area first can help diminish sensitivity.
- If you are an extremely sensitive individual, you may wish to purchase topical numbing agents.

- Make sure your injection fluid is room temperature or slightly warmer to lessen discomfort. A trick for warming medication is to roll the vial between your hands gently or hold the vial in your cupped hands and warm it with your breath. NEVER warm your medications in the microwave.

- Always flick the syringe to remove any large air bubbles. This will ensure you inject the full dosage of medication or as close as you can come to doing so. Hold the syringe with the needle pointing to the ceiling, wait for the bubbles to rise to the needle and then push them out by depressing the plunger so that the least amount of medication is lost through the needle tip.

- Never inject if pulling back on the plunger draws blood into the syringe. Withdraw the needle, apply pressure to stop any oozing and try injecting in a different spot. These injections should be either subcutaneous (just beneath the skin) or intramuscular (into the muscle), NOT intravenous (into the blood vessel).

- If you must inject your medications intramuscularly, a warm and relaxed muscle makes the injection less painful. Icing the area helps to numb the skin but a warm muscle accepts the injection more easily, so try both to find which works best for you. Warming the muscle and then icing the skin can be tricky, but can be accomplished to a certain extent.

Different Variations in Cycles

Although you will use the same medications as other couples, the length of time these medications are used and the timing of them can vary greatly. You may be concerned if your cycle is being run much differently than what you have read online, in books or have heard from your cycle buddies. Please realize that numerous protocols (treatment plans) exist for in vitro fertilization cycles and your diagnosis and previous cycles (if any) will influence which protocol your physician chooses.

Some cycles are termed long protocols because the gonadotropin-releasing hormone agonist (suppression medication) is started mid-cycle or following menses of the previous menstrual cycle, and continued until the hCG trigger shot is given. With the long protocol you begin with the GnRHa (suppression medication) and then add in the gonadotropin (stimulation medication) so that eventually you are administering two different medications in the same day. Some clinics will incorporate oral contraceptive pretreatment into a long protocol (in fact, oral contraceptives may be used in combination with any protocol), meaning you would begin taking birth control pills prior to starting the GnRHa—sometimes even months before.

Oral contraceptives improve the response to the stimulation medication and prevent ovulation by inhibiting the surge of luteinizing hormone (LH). Use of oral contraceptives also reduces the risk of forming functional cysts of the ovary that commonly occur with GnRHa use, especially with use over an extended period of time as with a long protocol. Oral contraceptives also eliminate the risk of beginning an IVF cycle following any spontaneous pregnancy of which you are unaware. Finally, oral contraceptives allow the clinic to schedule the egg retrieval to an exact date in advance because your RE completely controls the timing of your cycle.

Early cessation protocols begin GnRHa (suppression medication) administration mid-cycle of the previous menstrual cycle and continue until it is time to begin the stimulation medication. The gonadotropin (stimulation medication) is then taken until the hCG trigger shot. Typically, adequate suppression is achieved and a lower dose of the gonadotropin is required during the stimulation phase. With this protocol, you only administer one type of medication each day throughout your IVF cycle.

Short or flare protocols entail only a brief administration of GnRHa and "jump start" stimulation. The gonadotropin-releasing hormone agonist (suppression medication) is started on Day 2 of the cycle and then the stimulation medication is started one day later with both medications being continued until the hCG trigger shot. Because there is initial stimulation from the GnRHa, this protocol can boost follicle production in a poor responder (as can the use of oral contraceptives). One concern is the elevation of luteinizing hormone (LH) associated with microflare protocols. Although a small amount of LH is required for follicle growth and estrogen production, exposure to an excessive amount of LH can impair the quality of the egg and embryo. With a short or flare protocol, you start with a single medication and the next day add in a second medication (the gonadotropin) so that you are administering two different medications until you receive your hCG trigger shot.

"He who labors in any great or laudable undertaking has his fatigues first supported by hope, and afterward rewarded by joy."—*Samuel Johnson*

The dosage of the suppression medication also varies from patient to patient and may be changed during the course of an IVF cycle depending on how your body responds. Remember, your RE is trying to prevent ovulation by inhibiting the luteinizing hormone (LH) surge. However, the amount of GnRHa needed to prevent the LH surge is not known. Current dosages are based on studies done to determine the amount of GnRHa needed to give complete suppression in prostate cancer patients because no studies currently provide a minimum dose needed to prevent the LH surge during an IVF cycle. Therefore, it is not uncommon for the GnRHa dosage to be tweaked once your body demonstrates a response. Should your cycle be quite different from that of other IVFers, have faith that your RE is experienced and has chosen the best protocol for your given diagnosis and your response to the medications.

Timing Your Medications

It is important to be consistent with timing your medications. Choose a time that allows you to inject or sniff your medication at the same time each day or within an hour of that time. Should you be significantly delayed or completely miss your dose, contact your clinic immediately for instructions. Ovulation may occur with a missed dose and continuing the medication is fruitless as there will not be any eggs for your RE to retrieve. If this happens, don't beat yourself up over it. We are all human and make mistakes. Take it as a hard-learned lesson and forge forward.

Tips for Remembering Your Medications

Take your medications at the same time you do another daily activity. If you have a favorite show you never miss, or if you always brush your teeth right before bed, timing your medications to these events will help you to remember better. Leave your medications in plain sight or, if you wish to maintain privacy (as at work), create a small card to leave sitting out that will spark your memory (sticky notes or business cards work great and are easily overlooked by coworkers as normal office paraphernalia).

Monitoring for Suppression

In general, the suppression phase begins with the first dose of the gonadotropin-releasing hormone agonist (suppression medication) and ends when blood tests and an ultrasound exam show you are sufficiently suppressed, at which time the stimulation phase begins. Many women will have a period at the end of their suppression phase but many will not, depending on the protocol they are following. Your RE will perform a vaginal ultrasound prior to starting the stimulation medications to check for functional cysts that may have developed during GnRHa use. If several cysts or even a single large cyst has formed, your protocol may change or your cycle may be canceled to prevent complications down the line. Try not to lose heart if your cycle is canceled or extended. This is a very precise undertaking and time and care must be taken at all phases to help you reach your goal of parenthood.

Water, Water and More Water

It is extremely important to maintain adequate water intake to help reduce the risk of ovarian hyperstimulation syndrome (OHSS), a life threatening condition that can occur with the use of medications that stimulate the ovaries to produce multiple follicles. Prevention starts now and entails drinking plenty of water and avoiding excessively salty foods.

Why Some Clinics Skip Suppression

New IVF protocols are constantly emerging to improve pregnancy rates and lower complication rates. Some clinics now omit the suppression phase of an in vitro cycle. During medicated suppression, drug therapy ensures that no egg will reach maturity or subsequently be released (ovulated). Protocols which exclude medicated suppression do not down regulate the ovaries and this can be of benefit in older women (typically forty years or older) or in those women known to be poor responders to gonadotropin medications (the medications which stimulate egg production). Oftentimes, older women do not recover well from ovarian suppression and therefore have suboptimal follicle production and egg quality. By omitting the suppression phase, there is no risk of medication side effects and often improved egg production and quality occurs.

"Look within. Within is the fountain of good, and it will ever bubble up if thou wilt ever dig."
—*Ancient saying*

The IVF Blues

Manipulation of normal hormone production during the suppression phase can bring on the IVF blues even if you are feeling quite optimistic at the start of your cycle. As estrogen levels fall to menopausal levels, the drop in estrogen can greatly affect energy levels, mood and enthusiasm. Headaches that are resistant to pain relievers often occur. Insomnia in the form of difficulty falling asleep, restless sleep or early morning waking also contributes to the blue hue of this phase.

Whether you readily notice it or not, you will find your emotions are much more unstable during the suppression phase. Irritability is a common complaint, as is tearfulness. You and your partner may find yourselves arguing more frequently, often over minor things.

HINT for WOMEN

Sleep, even if just a short nap, can help alleviate the headaches associated with the suppression phase.

HINT for GUYS

Small gestures can go a long way during this phase of your cycle. Flowers, a sweet card or a night out for just the two of you will remind your partner that her efforts are noted and appreciated. Something as simple as a hug and an "I love you" can make even the worse suppression day seem better.

You may also find your outlook less optimistic and feel the obstacles before you are too great to overcome. To feel less social and to withdraw from others at times is not uncommon, especially in regards to social gatherings. These changes occur slowly over the course of the suppression phase and will linger into the stimulation phase until estrogen levels begin to rise.

Knowing what potentially lies ahead for you physically and emotionally in the suppression phase can prepare you to deal with the side effects more effectively. Pamper yourself during this time and avoid situations that might evoke strong emotions (baby showers, in-laws staying with you, etc.). Remember, this is just a temporary phase you must pass through that will fade quickly enough. Surround yourself with positive energy and with people who are supportive and understanding. Music is a great way to moderate the mood swings associated with suppression; choose uplifting music to raise your spirits or soothing sounds to calm your nerves. Aromatherapy is also a wonderful way to pamper your mind and body as you cycle. Incorporate aromatherapy (lavender is wonderful for stress relief) by using scented bath oils or scented candles. Consider acupuncture treatments to deal with the elevated stress levels and avoid stressful situations as much as possible while feeling blue. And, even if you aren't a fan of writing, keep a journal that documents your journey to parenthood. Writing down the feelings and emotions you are experiencing often helps you deal with them better.

Overview of the Suppression Phase

- There is great variation regarding in vitro cycles but the general goal is to prevent your body from ovulating eggs before they can be retrieved.

- Your individual treatment plan will be based on your age and diagnosis as well as previous cycle outcomes.

- Be consistent with your medications. Take your medications at the same time each day or within an hour.

- You may experience some pretty nasty side effects, so remind yourself that this is only temporary and that you CAN make it to the next phase.

- Do not lose hope. It is common to feel overwhelmed by what lies ahead and to feel as though your cycle will be a failure. Your dropping estrogen level contributes significantly to feeling this way, and you will feel renewed hope during the stimulation phase as your estrogen level rises.

- Pamper yourself. This is a difficult undertaking and it is important to do special little things to maintain your focus and sanity!

- When/if your period arrives, celebrate. After so many months of dreading the arrival of Aunt Flo, you are finally happy to be seeing red! It marks the end of the suppression phase and allows you to shift gears toward growing follicles.

Chapter Eight

The Stimulation Phase

preparation...suppression...stimulation...egg retrieval...
embryo transfer...two week wait...and beyond

Grow, Follies, Grow!

During the stimulation phase, your body's energy goes into producing multiple, mature eggs. These are the eggs which will be retrieved in the next phase of your IVF cycle: the egg retrieval phase. Like many couples, you may begin counting the days of your cycle based on the start date of your stimulation phase rather than the start date of the suppression phase. Either is fine, as long as you are consistent and in synch with your clinic. If you were suppressed with medications, you will find your energy level and outlook improving greatly and your headaches dissipating as you progress through the stimulation phase. During this phase, fertility drugs called gonadotropins are used to stimulate the ovaries to produce multiple follicles.

FOLLICLES vs. EGGS

A follicle is an ovarian structure which contains the egg (oocyte) and a surrounding cell layer. The egg is aspirated from the follicle during egg retrieval.

Ultrasounds performed during the stimulation phase monitor the size and number of follicles within each ovary.

Often the stimulation phase will last twelve to sixteen days, but may be longer or shorter depending on your response to the medication. The gonadotropin medications used during this phase are one of two types: human menopausal gonadotropins (hMG) or recombinant gonadotropins.

Types of Stimulation Medications

	Recombinant Gonadotropin	Human Menopausal Gonadotropin
Origin	Produced from the isolated genes for human FSH. These genes are inserted into Chinese hamster ovary cells, which are then induced to produce high amounts of FSH. It is this FSH that is then purified for use.	Produced by isolating and purifying the hormones FSH and LH from the urine of postmenopausal women. These medications contain small amounts of urinary proteins, however there are no known cases of disease transmission through these medications.
Trade Name	• Gonal-F • Follistim • Fertinex • Bravelle These are referred to as follitropins.	• Repronex • Pergonal • Humegon These are referred to as menotropins.
Hormone	FSH only	FSH & LH

These medications are injectable and either contain both follicle-stimulating hormone (FSH) and luteinizing hormone (LH), or contain FSH only. The FSH is responsible for maturation of the ovarian follicles. Normally, the pituitary gland senses low estrogen levels and begins releasing FSH to stimulate follicular growth and development. As the follicles develop, they release estrogen. Under normal conditions, this increasing level of estrogen tells the pituitary gland to slow down FSH production so that only one egg comes to full maturity (it is possible for more than one egg to reach maturity, though, and this can result in twins, triplets, etc.). In the manipulated setting of an IVF cycle, stimulation medications containing FSH are injected, maintaining an elevated level of FSH regardless of the estrogen level. Your RE controls what your FSH level is through daily injections of the stimulation medications. Ultimately, this allows you to have multiple eggs that develop to full maturity in a single cycle; hence the term, controlled ovarian hyperstimulation.

The Endometrial Lining

As multiple follicles develop, the estrogen level begins to rise (the follicles produce estrogen). The rising estrogen level improves your mood and washes away the suppression blues. More importantly, the rising estrogen level causes proliferation or thickening of the endometrium (the layer of the inner uterus in which the embryo will implant). In general, the desired endometrial thickness is 8-13 mm, as measured by ultrasound. Often 11 mm is the thickness IVFers hope to achieve. A thickness less than 6 mm is a potential problem, as the embryo may fail to implant. A thickness greater than 15 mm may reduce the chances for a successful pregnancy. Although IVFers often get caught up in counting follicles, the endometrial lining thickness is important to the successful outcome of a cycle. Too thin or too thick of a lining lowers the chances of the embryo attaching.

Monitoring and testing are the mainstays of the stimulation phase. Blood tests will be done to monitor your estradiol (E2) and luteinizing hormone (LH) levels. Rising E2 levels will guide your physician with gonadotropin (stimulation medication) administration, and low LH levels will prevent premature ovulation prior to egg retrieval. Remember, if you ovulate, there is no egg left within the follicle and therefore no egg available to retrieve.

ESTROGEN vs. ESTRADIOL

Estrogen refers to both natural estrogen hormones within the body as well as estrogen products used in medications. There are three forms of estrogen in your body: E1, E2 and E3.

- E1—estrone, produced in ovaries and fat tissue; main estrogen in postmenopausal women
- E2—estradiol, produced in ovaries; main estrogen in pre-menopausal women; monitored during IVF cycle
- E3—estriol, weakest of the three estrogens and produced from other estrogens

When discussing an in vitro cycle, estrogen is often used interchangeably with estradiol for ease of discussion.

The further into the stimulation phase you progress, the more frequent blood draws will become. It is during this stage that you may develop noticeable bruising at the blood draw sites.

HINT for WOMEN

Wear long-sleeved shirts to hide bruising. This can eliminate the curious stares and questions from concerned friends or co-workers.

Monitoring Your Follicles

Monitoring will also involve vaginal probe ultrasound examinations typically beginning a couple of days into the stimulation phase and lasting until the day of the hCG trigger shot. As you progress, your physician will monitor you more frequently (daily in some cases) until your endometrial lining reaches an adequate thickness and the majority of follicles reach the appropriate size for egg retrieval. Each RE may have her own guidelines, but a general guideline for lining thickness is 11 mm. For follicle size, it is 15-18 mm.

Reduce Activity Levels

As the ovary enlarges, it is more prone to ovarian torsion, a situation in which the ovary twists on itself, cutting off its own blood supply. Heavy exercise, strenuous activity or jarring motions increase the risk of torsion and rupture of follicles.

It is important to remember that ultrasound provides limited information as far as follicle number. Follicles that are nestled behind each other may appear as a single follicle on ultrasound. More often than not, more follicles are present than estimated. It is also important to remember that follicles greater than 15mm in diameter can contain eggs at different maturity levels and some follicles may contain no egg at all. Follicles which measure less than 14 mm typically have immature eggs that are difficult to fertilize. For this reason, the combined results of blood testing and ultrasound monitoring give the best chance for the greatest number of mature eggs to be retrieved.

"True hope dwells on the possible, even when life seems to be a plot written by someone who wants to see how much adversity we can overcome."
—*Walter Anderson*

Poor vs. High Responders

Your response to the stimulation medications can vary greatly from a poor response with few follicles produced to a strong response with many follicles produced. You may hear women comment that they are either poor responders or high responders depending on the number of follicles produced and the E2 level reached. Although there will be variation from clinic to clinic and lab to lab regarding what qualifies as a poor response or a high response, the following chart provides a general guideline:

	Poor Responder	Mid-Responder	High Responder
E2 on day of hCG trigger	<500	500–1500	>1500
Development of mature eggs	lower	same	Same (lower w/E2>3000)
Dividing embryos	same	same	same
Pregnancy rate	lower	same	Same (lower w/E2>3000)

If you are a poor responder, your response to the stimulation medication is suboptimal, as is follicle development. You will likely produce fewer than four mature eggs or will fail to reach a peak E2 level of at least 500. Often you hear of poor responders producing only one to two follicles and, in some cases, no follicles. Typically, the number of mature eggs retrieved is low because of the decreased number of follicles, and the resulting embryos often divide at similar rates as the embryos of women who have a normal response or a high response to gonadotropin stimulation. Pregnancy rates are lower with poor responders because the minimum E2 level required for implantation is not reached. Mid-responders in the above table refer to those patients who have a normal response to the stimulation medications and produce an adequate number of follicles while maintaining an E2 level within the clinic's "target range". Mid-responders provide a point of reference when comparing poor and high responders. If you are a high responder, your body has a strong response to the stimulation medications. You will produce many follicles and will have pregnancy rates similar to mid-responders, except when the E2 level is greater than 3000. With an E2 level greater than 3000, you will develop a greater number of small to mid-sized follicles, but more follicles will contain immature eggs. You will have a lower pregnancy rate, as compared to mid-responders, due to poor implantation since uterine receptivity is decreased with high E2 levels. It is important to realize that as a poor responder or high responder you can still achieve pregnancy.

Why the concern over your response to stimulation medications? If you respond either poorly or excessively during this phase, you will face unique problems with your cycle, problems which may be in addition to the ones you already face. If you are a poor responder, your RE may consider one of the following: (1) high-dose gonadotropin cycle; (2) low-dose gonadotropin-releasing hormone agonist (GnRHa) or omitted suppression phase cycle; (3) co-treatment with growth hormone. Conversely, if you have a significantly increased response to gonadotropin medications and produce high levels of estradiol, your RE will typically recommend low-dose gonadotropins.

HINT for GUYS

Help out more with household chores and take on the more strenuous responsibilities at home.

Ovarian Hyperstimulation Syndrome

One of the most worrisome potential complicatons of the stimulation phase is the development of ovarian hyperstimulation syndrome—commonly called OHSS. Ovarian hyperstimulation syndrome can occur following the use of gonadotropin medications and in its severe form can be life-threatening. It is not something to be taken lightly and will be at the forefront of your RE's mind as she monitors your E2 levels.

Ovarian hyperstimulation syndrome is divided into two types: mild-moderate and severe.

- Mild-Moderate: Occurs in 10 to 20 percent of cycles; some discomfort but typically resolves spontaneously in a couple of days
- Severe: Occurs in 1 percent of cycles; can result in chest and abdominal fluid build-up, ovarian torsion, blood clots, kidney damage, electrolyte imbalance and severe pain; typically requires hospitalization for monitoring and occasionally drainage of fluid; lasts approximately one to two weeks; IVFers with an E2 level greater than 3000 pg/ml and greater than thirty follicles on ultrasound are at increased risk of developing severe OHSS[14]

You and your partner should be familiar with the signs and symptoms of OHSS and report any concerns to your physician immediately.

Signs and Symptoms of OHSS

You may experience abdominal discomfort, nausea, vomiting, weight gain, decreased urine production, shortness of breath, difficulty breathing, or pelvic pain.

If your RE feels ovarian hyperstimulation syndrome is likely to occur based on the trend of your rising E2 level, she may decide to coast you for a few days. Coasting entails stopping the stimulation medication and withholding the hCG trigger shot until the E2 level decreases. Coasting is commonly initiated when the E2 level reaches 2500 to 3000. After stopping the medication, the E2 level will continue to rise for one to days and the follicles will continue to increase in diameter. Coasting should be done for fewer than four days as a decrease in implantation and pregnancy rates is associated with coasting for greater than four days.[15] Since hCG is a triggering factor for the development of OHSS, the hCG trigger shot will typically not be given until the E2 level drops below 3000. Should OHSS occur following the hCG trigger shot, you may not proceed to embryo transfer following a successful egg retrieval. Rather, you will wait for the OHSS to resolve and undergo a frozen embryo transfer at a later date. If your RE feels you are at risk for developing severe OHSS, the cycle may be canceled. Subsequent cycles may be altered to avoid such an exaggerated response, allowing you to proceed through an entire cycle.

Risk Factors for OHSS

- Polycystic ovarian syndrome (PCOS)
- Age less than thirty-five
- Lean body type
- High E2 level
- Human chorionic gonadotropin (hCG)

The hCG Trigger Shot

Once the majority of follicles reach the appropriate range in size, the hCG trigger shot is given. Since only mature eggs can be fertilized, the hCG trigger shot is administered to induce maturation of the egg. In an IVF cycle, the hCG is dispensed as a powder and must be mixed with dilute (normal saline) to allow intramuscular (IM) injection. It is important to inject all of the liquid in the syringe directly into the muscle.

---

hCG trigger dose range is 2,000-10,000 IU

The hCG trigger shot is exactly timed to allow for egg retrieval thirty-six hours later. This provides ample time for the eggs to fully mature without actually being released (ovulated) from the follicle.

hCG SPOTTING

You may experience spotting following the hCG trigger shot. Always notify your physician of bleeding, even if it is just mild spotting.

The stimulation medications have potential side effects, which include abdominal or pelvic pain (often due to the enlarging ovaries), weight gain, nausea, vomiting, breast discomfort, and abnormal uterine bleeding. Because these are injectable medications, it is also possible to experience pain, swelling, itching, and/or irritation at the injection site, as well as develop a localized infection if sterile techniques are not employed.

The Final Days of Stimulation

The stimulation phase cumulates with three orders from your RE: (1) administer your hCG trigger shot at a specific time to allow for egg retrieval in thirty-six to thirty-seven hours, (2) begin your oral antibiotic, (3) have sexual intercourse. Take your time injecting the hCG as it is important to get all of the medication into the muscle. The buttocks are the preferred spot of injection. Make sure to begin your antibiotics to protect against infection following the egg retrieval procedure. Make a romantic evening for yourselves so that your sexual interlude is one of passion and love. You will have a thirty-six hour break from injections and monitoring—enjoy them to the fullest. If intercourse just isn't a possibility, your partner must take matters into his own hands. Ejaculation the night of the hCG trigger is important to ensure the best possible semen sample on the day of egg retrieval.

Overview of the Stimulation Phase

- The goal of the stimulation phase is to produce multiple, mature eggs without over-stimulating the ovaries and to thicken the endometrial lining such that an embryo is able to attach.

- Remember, cycles can vary greatly from couple to couple, so do not be alarmed if your cycle seems to be quite different from someone else's.

- Watch for the signs and symptoms of OHSS: bloating, pelvic pain, dwindling urine output, nausea, vomiting, difficulty breathing, and/or shortness of breath.

- Don't lose faith if it takes longer to reach the best follicle size and endometrial lining thickness than you anticipated. This is not a race but rather a steady climb towards the desired results.

- Follow instructions closely the night you trigger so that your egg retrieval is timed appropriately.

- Make your trigger night a love romp rather than a calculated necessity.

Chapter Nine

Egg Retrieval

preparation…suppression…stimulation…egg retrieval…
embryo transfer…two week wait…and beyond

Beautiful Eggs Become Beautiful Embies

Your hard work finally pays off as you enter the egg retrieval phase. Thirty-six hours prior to your egg retrieval, oral antibiotics are started to reduce the risk of infection, as this an invasive procedure. As with any outpatient procedure, food and liquid intake is restricted several hours prior to egg retrieval. It is important to arrive at the designated time (usually thirty to sixty minutes before your actual egg retrieval procedure) so that your clinic has ample time to get you prepped.

HINT for COUPLES

Give yourselves plenty of time to make your appointment in the event of bad weather or an accident on the road. Know at least one alternate route to the clinic in case there is a problem with traffic or construction.

The Egg Retrieval Procedure

Remember, you will not have your partner in the room with you as they must provide a fresh semen sample to be used for fertilization of any retrieved eggs. Use relaxation techniques to lessen any anxiety you might experience before the procedure actually begins. A light sedative or anesthetic may be used, but some physicians have their patients remain awake throughout the procedure. If this concerns you, ask for sedation to make the procedure more tolerable and to lessen your anxiety.

HINT for WOMEN

Bring a little baggie for the ride home. Some women may become nauseated from the medications used during the ER procedure.

In general, a transvaginal ultrasound probe is used to provide images of the follicles within your ovaries. A long, hollow needle is threaded alongside the ultrasound probe and pushed through the vaginal wall into the follicle. Each follicle is aspirated in succession, with the contents of each follicle placed into a test tube and handed to the embryologist. The embryologist then transfers the contents of each test tube to a small, flat dish, called a Petri dish. Each Petri dish is examined under the microscope to identify if the egg is present and to determine its suitability for fertilization. Remember, only mature eggs can be fertilized.

In uncomplicated cases, the egg retrieval procedure will take less than thirty minutes. If there are a large number of follicles present or if the follicles are difficult to reach, the procedure may take longer than anticipated. It is not uncommon to have some light spotting following egg retrieval due to puncture of the vaginal wall.

HINT for WOMEN

Wear a panty liner in case you have mild spotting after your retrieval.

Possible Complications of Egg Retrieval

If a small blood vessel is punctured during the procedure, it is possible to have cramping and pelvic pain after the procedure. Alert your physician to these symptoms as they can be treated with pain medications. Heavy bleeding or severe pain may indicate a more serious complication, such as puncture of a surrounding organ, and requires immediate attention. To date, there is no evidence to suggest that the procedure of egg retrieval damages the ovary in any way.

Understanding Terminology

- EGGS are retrieved
- A fertilized egg is a ZYGOTE
- A zygote develops into an EMBRYO

Semen Sample Collection

At the same time the eggs are retrieved, your partner will be required to provide a fresh semen sample in the clinic's collection room. Frozen sperm may also be utilized for fertilization, in which case your partner does not need to provide a sample. If you have followed your RE's guidelines, it should have been at least thirty-six hours since the last ejaculation (this gives the best quality sample possible and can vary from clinic to clinic, with some recommending forty-eight hours). Make sure your partner is aware that this collection can be much more stressful and nerve-racking than the previous collection for the semen analysis. The clinical nature and time constraints of the collection as well as your partner's concern for you often make this task difficult, yet a good sample is important. The stress associated with providing this sample has been shown to decrease semen quality[16], so he should plan ahead and incorporate relaxation techniques such as deep breathing and visualization to help ease the stress of this collection. Sperm from this fresh sample are then mixed with the eggs within several hours of retrieval to allow fertilization to occur.

Fertilization Methods

Fertilization can occur in one of two ways:

1. **Standard insemination,** in which the egg and sperm are placed close to each other within the growth media and the sperm are allowed to fertilize the egg by normal mechanisms of attachment and penetration (as would happen in unassisted conception). This technique is used if you and your partner have no egg quality issues or male factor issues.

2. **Micromanipulation techniques,** including intracytoplasmic sperm injection, sub-zonal insemination and partial zona dissection.

   a. **Intracytoplasmic sperm injection (ICSI)**—With this technique, a single isolated sperm is drawn up into a specially designed pipette. The pipette is inserted into the egg's center (the cytoplasm) and the sperm is released. This technique may be used if you and your partner have severe male factor issues or egg quality issues. Intracytoplasmic sperm injection may also be used if you have had poor fertilization results with previous cycles. This is the newest of the three forms of micromanipulation to aid fertilization and brings great hope for many couples.

b. **Sub-zonal Insemination (SUZI)**—With this technique, an opening is made in the zona pellucida (thick outer shell of ovum) and the sperm is injected between the egg and zona pellucida.

c. **Partial Zona Dissection (PZD)**—With this technique, the zona pellucida is opened to allow sperm to enter more easily. The amount of sperm entering the oocyte is not controlled as with SUZI.

Once the egg and sperm have been combined, they then find their way to the incubator where optimal conditions facilitate growth and development of the embryo. Your embryos will be watched closely and you will receive updates on their progress over the next few days.

HINT for COUPLES

Ask for a picture of your embryos and give them a pet name. This is a wonderful keepsake and helps you connect with your embies as a part of both of you rather than just as a medical term.

Immediately following the egg retrieval procedure, you will be taken to a different room where you are allowed to awaken from the sedation. Like many women, you may feel quite sore following the procedure as medications wear off and you will find it most comfortable to rest at home for the remainder of the day. It is not uncommon to be lightheaded or drowsy following egg retrieval, so use caution. You will not be able to drive home, so make sure either your loved one or a friend can get you home safely. The day of egg retrieval also marks the first day you begin taking your progesterone. There are two ways progesterone can be taken, either injection directly into the muscle or vaginal suppository.

Taking Progesterone

Progesterone in oil (PIO) is administered via injection directly into the muscle tissue and can be quite uncomfortable. The PIO needle is larger than the needles previously used in your cycle and the oil suspension tends to sit in the muscle, causing soreness and formation of lumps. Icing the area prior to injecting alleviates some of the discomfort, and gently massaging the muscle after injection helps dissipate the oil suspension. Soak in a warm bath or apply a heating pad to the injection site following injection of the PIO to lessen your discomfort.

Progesterone in oil takes longer to inject because it is such a thick fluid. Take your time and make sure you get the dose fully injected. Alternate the sites of injection to keep from getting too sore in any one area and always administer these injections daily, even if they are painful, as progesterone helps support early pregnancy.

"Each difficult moment has the potential to open my eyes and open my heart."—*Myla Kabat-Zinn*

Progesterone can also be administered as a vaginal suppository. It is dispensed as a small, white oval pill inserted into the vagina where it is directly absorbed. Because the vaginal suppository works more directly on the uterus and has less of an effect on blood levels as compared to progesterone in oil, your RE is less likely to monitor your progesterone through blood draws. Lying flat following placement of the suppository will minimize leakage of the medication. It is a good idea to wear a panty liner if you need to be up and moving around shortly after placing the suppository. If you are sexually active while using the progesterone suppositories, place the progesterone after intercourse to minimize leakage.

Inform Your Doctor

In the event you become pregnant, notify your obstetrician that you are using the progesterone suppository. This will avoid unnecessary treatment for a yeast infection—the white suppository may look suspect and be misinterpreted as yeast.

Regardless of how you administer the progesterone, the goal is to supplement your body's progesterone levels in order to support the pregnancy you may well achieve very soon. Although the exact mechanism by which the progesterone works is not clearly understood, there are several theories. One theory is that medications used during the suppression phase limit luteinizing hormone, which normally supports progesterone production. Another is that the egg retrieval process disrupts the cells that normally produce progesterone. A third theory is that supplemental progesterone is needed to bring the ratio of estrogen (which is greatly elevated during an IVF cycle) and progesterone closer to the normal ratio seen in unassisted conception. Whatever the mechanism, there is improvement in pregnancy rates with supplemental progesterone.

Progesterone is continued into the first trimester of pregnancy, but each RE has her own guidelines for how many weeks the medication is continued. Some will stop the progesterone after just a few weeks and others will continue progesterone for the entire first trimester of pregnancy. If you face PIO injections, this can seem an eternity. Try as many tricks and techniques as possible to lessen the discomfort of these injections. Remind yourself of the wonderful possibilities before you and focus your attention on your embies as they grow.

Overview of Egg Retrieval

- With the prospect of a needle puncturing your ovaries numerous times looming ahead, the egg retrieval procedure can make even the calmest woman anxious. Express your desires for sedation during egg retrieval and visualize your tiny baby, waiting to be created.

- Not all follicles show up on ultrasound, and not all follicles contain eggs, so try to remain realistic in your expectations and avoid comparing your egg count to fellow IVFers. Each egg brings you closer to your dream, but quality counts just as much as quantity.

- Take it easy following your procedure. It is invasive and the medications used during your egg retrieval can affect you for some time after the procedure.

- Make this journey personal by giving your embryos special pet names and cheer them on as you wait for your embryo transfer. They are very much a part of you both and making this connection can soften the clinical aspect of IVF.

- Be faithful with your progesterone injections even if they are quite painful or difficult to get through. Progesterone helps maintain a pregnancy and in the end, all the discomforts of a cycle are well worth it!

- Celebrate this accomplishment. It has been a difficult path with more difficulties yet to come, but rejoice for each completed phase and prepare for the challenges that are still ahead.

Chapter Ten

Embryo Transfer

preparation…suppression…stimulation…egg retrieval…
embryo transfer…two week wait…and beyond

Time to Bring Your Embies Home!

Embryo transfer is the procedure by which your reproductive endocrinologist places your embryos within your uterus or your zygotes within the Fallopian tube in the case of a zygote intrafallopian transfer (ZIFT).

Updates on Your Embryos

On the first day following your egg retrieval, you will receive updates from your clinic. The first update will entail your fertilization results and possibly the division number of your embryos, if the call comes late in the day. Your fertilization results may vary greatly from other infertility couples and from cycle to cycle. It is best to prepare for the worst and hope for the best. Expecting 100 percent fertilization is unrealistic. As we IVFers always say, "It only takes one!" There is always hope as long as one of your eggs fertilizes and begins to develop as an embryo.

Subsequent updates will entail how many embryos are still viable and how much division has occurred. Most likely at least some embryos will stop developing, with an increasing chance of embryo loss the longer the laboratory incubation period lasts.

Embryo Cell Division

A general timeline for embryo development/division follows this scenario: Day 0 is your retrieval day → most Day 2 embryos will have 2-4 cells, if not more → typically, Day 3 embryos will have 6-8 cells, if not more → Day 4 embryos have divided enough to contain 16-32 cells or more (termed a morula) → Day 5 embryos will have 60-160 cells, or so many it is impossible to count the individual cells (termed a blastocyst) → by or on Day 6, the zona pellucida is lost and the embryo is capable of implantation.[17] The rate of development is closely correlated with the potential for the embryo to survive, but it is possible for some embryos to develop more slowly and still go on to be a term pregnancy. Obviously, severely lagging embryos are more likely to stop developing than rapidly dividing embryos.

"Hope is a waking dream."—*Aristotle*

Embryo Grading

In addition to the number of cells present, the quality of the embryo also gives clues to its viability (ability to survive). A small amount of fragmentation (ejection of some of the cytoplasm from the dividing cell) is considered normal, but some embryos may suffer with excessive fragmentation. By combining the cell number and quality, your embryologist will grade your embryo. There is no standard for the grading of embryos and many clinics have their own system for denoting which embryos have the best chance of leading to a viable pregnancy. Some clinics may give the best embryos the lowest number (0 or 1), and other clinics may give the best embryos the highest number (3 or 4), so always check with your clinic to learn what system they use to grade embryos. There is a push to develop a universal grading system to help embryologists choose the best embryos for transfer, but to date there are no set guidelines for clinics to follow. Again, a poor rating for an embryo does not doom it as many couples have been blessed with babies who started out labeled as a "poor grade" embryo.

Updates on your embies will be something along the lines of "You have five embryos: two 8 cell embryos and three 10 cell embryos, with one of the 8 cell embryos and two of the 10 cell embryos showing large amounts of fragmentation," or, "You have two excellent 16 cell embryos, two good 12 cell embryos and one poor 10 cell embryo." Your clinic may use letters or numbers, or a combination of the two to denote the embryo grade. Your clinic may also simply describe your embies as excellent, good or poor. If you are unsure what the assigned grade actually means, don't be afraid to ask. IVFers tend to cheer their embies on during these first few days of development, and it can really ease your mind to hear how they are progressing while you wait for transfer day to arrive.

Pre-implantation Genetic Diagnosis

Like some couples, you may opt for pre-implantation genetic diagnosis (PGD) to aid in the selection of those embryos to be transferred or cryopreserved. This procedure is a diagnostic tool that allows determination of the embryo's genetic composition while still only at the four to eight cell stage of development. In order to perform pre-implantation genetic diagnosis, one to two cells must be removed from each embryo considered for transfer or cryopreservation. Because this is invasive, there is the risk of damaging the developing embryo such that it stops dividing. Pre-implantation genetic diagnosis testing is performed and embryos are allowed to continue developing, with results coming back before the time of embryo transfer.

Pre-implantation genetic diagnosis involves evaluating the chromosomal composition (called aneuploidy testing) and determining the absence or presence of specific genes. Not all twenty-three chromosome pairs are evaluated, but PGD allows for the detection of chromosomally linked conditions such as Down syndrome and Turner's syndrome. Testing for the presence or absence of specific genes provides valuable information for couples known to be carriers of genes responsible for diseases such as cystic fibrosis, Duchenne muscular dystrophy, hemophilia type A and Tay-Sachs disease. It is possible to determine the sex of the embryo, but the use of PGD for gender selection is a very controversial subject.

If you and your partner have a family history of a genetic disorder or are known to be carriers of certain diseases, or if you are older than thirty-five years of age, you may wish to consider testing your embryos. Pre-implantation genetic diagnosis allows the embryologist to determine the genetic composition of an embryo at an early stage and influences her choice regarding which embryo(s) to transfer. This can negate the need for genetic testing during pregnancy, which may require you and your partner to make a very difficult ethical decision concerning carrying your pregnancy to term.

Assisted Hatching

Depending on your age, diagnosis and previous IVF cycle outcomes, your embryos may undergo what is called assisted hatching. The zona pellucida (thick shell surrounding the early embryo) is typically lost by or on Day 6, allowing the embryo to break out of the shell and attach itself to the uterine wall. In some instances, the embryo needs help breaking through this shell in order to implant.

Assisted hatching involves creating a gap in the zona pellucida, thereby improving implantation rates should you have factors such as:

- Advanced age in woman (greater than 37-38 years of age)
- Elevated Day 3 FSH (decreased ovarian reserve, egg quality and quantity concerns)
- Excessively fragmented embryos
- Embryos with excessively thick zona pellucida
- Previous cycle failures

Assisted hatching can be performed in one of three ways: (1) use of a specialized pipette to create a mechanical "tear," (2) use of Tyrode's solution to chemically create a gap, (3) use of a laser. Assisted hatching is a very precise technique. A hole made too large or too small may hinder implantation rather than facilitate it. Regardless of the technique used to create the gap, the end result is the same.

Finally, after anxiously awaiting each status report on your embies and cheering them on, embryo transfer day arrives and it is time to bring them home. The wait time from egg retrieval to embryo transfer will vary and is dependent on many factors, including age, diagnosis, development of embryos and physician preference. It is possible to transfer embryos as early as Day 1 and as late as Day 6. Many reproductive endocrinologists are moving toward Day 5 transfers in an attempt to lower the risk of multiple gestations (twins, triplets, etc.), because fewer embryos are transferred with a blastocyst transfer (Day 5–Day 6). However, not all embryos are capable of sustaining life in the artificial laboratory setting even though they might do well in the natural environment of the woman's uterus. In this instance, a Day 3 transfer is typically performed.

Day 3 vs. Day 5 Transfer

There are pros and cons for Day 3 and Day 5 transfers and it is important to discuss your transfer with your doctor so that you feel comfortable with your decision. Most often, a larger number of embryos are transferred on Day 3 because less growth and differentiation have occurred and it is more challenging to choose which embryos are of the highest quality. This puts you at much greater risk of having a multiple gestation pregnancy. Although many IVFers welcome the idea of twins or triplets, the risks and complications of a multiple gestation pregnancy should be taken seriously. The increased risk of premature labor and long-term issues preemies face, as well as complications from pregnancy itself, can be life threatening or debilitating for both the mother and the babies. Should you and your partner transfer a larger number of embryos on Day 3, you may also need to face the difficult decision of selective reduction, should all embryos implant. It is important to remember that the goal of IVF is to achieve pregnancy, not to achieve twins or triplets. On the upside, if your embryos would not survive in the lab for more than three days, you have a viable option for achieving pregnancy with a Day 3 transfer.

With a Day 5 transfer (called a blast or blastocyst transfer), you and your partner may run the risk of losing all your embryos by waiting the five days. Not all labs have the same experience maintaining embryos in the lab for five days and the quantity and quality of embryos may be affected by this. Typically, only one to two embryos are transferred on Day 5, greatly reducing the risk of triplets or quadruplets and, since more differentiation has occurred, it may be easier for the embryologist to choose the best quality embryos.

The Embryo Transfer Procedure

Regardless on which day you transfer your embryos, the procedure is the same. Both you and your partner will be in the same room and you will be asked to lie on your back as you would for a Pap smear. Your RE will place a vaginal speculum to allow easier passage of the catheter. An ultrasound probe will be placed on your abdomen to guide placement of the catheter. Embryo transfer uses a specially designed catheter to place human embryos directly into the uterine cavity. The embryos are carried into the uterine cavity in a fluid called transfer medium, with the catheter transferring both the media and the embryo(s) into the uterus. The catheter and speculum are then slowly removed.

HINT for COUPLES

Ask for a photo of your embryo transfer ultrasound. The bright area is the fluid in which your embies are floating.

The embryo transfer procedure is much less painful than the egg retrieval procedure. There may be some discomfort from the use of a speculum or manipulation of the uterus as your RE achieves optimal catheter placement. Embryo transfer basically feels like a Pap smear and only takes a few minutes to complete. Embryo transfer is often more difficult if you have a stenotic cervical os (a narrowing of the opening of the cervix) or an unusually angled uterus. In this instance, there may be more spotting due to increased manipulation or tight passage of the catheter through the narrowed opening of the cervix.

The number of transferred embryos will be determined by the age and medical diagnoses of you and your partner, embryo quality and quantity, the day of transfer (Day 3 vs. Day 5), you and your partner's wishes and the advice of your reproductive endocrinologist. The embryo(s) are placed relative to the uterine fundus, requiring a gentle touch by your RE. Embryos placed too high in the uterus or too low in the uterus may be a significant contributing factor to the low implantation rates of in vitro. The catheter will be closely inspected following the transfer to ensure no embryos remain in the catheter. Any embryos not transferred will be monitored until they are cryopreserved (if you have chosen to freeze your remaining embryos).

Cryopreservation of Embryos

Cryopreservation is the process of freezing, storing and thawing embryos for future use. Embryo cryopreservation began in 1948 with the accidental successful cryopreservation of fowl sperm. Scientists mislabeled some experimental freezing solutions and accidentally used glycerol rather than another compound. Since then, cryopreservation has had the greatest impact in the field of reproduction. Procedures for human embryo freezing were developed in 1984 and only went into widespread use in the late 1980s.

In addition to preservation of viable embryos not transferred during an IVF cycle, cryopreservation may also be used for the following reasons:

- Risk of or impending severe ovarian hyperstimulation syndrome (OHSS)
- Poor quality endometrium (thin uterine lining)

- Intermenstrual bleeding
- Development of a condition (cysts, hydrosalpinx, etc.) during the cycle that requires additional treatment after retrieval, but before transfer is done.

You and your partner will be notified of the number of embryos to be frozen and often what stage of development the embryos are at prior to freezing. For cryopreservation, the embryos are placed into straws or vials containing cryoprotectants (antifreeze). Cryoprotectants help prevent the build up of salts, as water crystallizes during freezing. They are then placed into a special freezer that uses a slow and controlled rate of cooling. During cooling, cells dehydrate, ice forms and water is removed from the cells. This all happens gradually as high levels of salts and the ice crystals themselves could hurt the cells during freezing or thawing. This slow cooling process is continued until a temperature of -32.8°F/-36ºC is reached. At that point, embryos are rapidly cooled by a plunge into liquid nitrogen (-320.8°F/-196ºC). The embryos are then placed in liquid nitrogen storage tanks. The entire freezing process takes several hours. It is important to bear in mind that not all embryos are candidates for cryopreservation. If the embryo is not of good enough quality, it will not be frozen. This guideline is in place as studies have shown high quality embryos are much more likely to survive freezing and thawing. Embryos with slow development or significant fragmentation will not be preserved. Although rates will vary, typically 20 to 30 percent of embryos will make it to cryopreservation. Factors influencing the number of embryos which make it to cryopreservation include the number of eggs retrieved, the number of eggs fertilized, egg quality and lab skill.[18] To date, there is no evidence to suggest that extended periods of storage affect the viability of the embryo. You may receive a bill from the embryologist for this service and for the first year of embryo storage, which averages $300. Insurance companies may not cover this expense so be prepared to pay out of pocket if need be.

If you and your partner undergo frozen embryo transfer, you will use your previously frozen embryos (affectionately termed ice babies, frosties and totsicles in the infertility community) for transfer. The thawing process is much quicker than the freezing process, at about thirty to forty-five minutes. When embryos come out of the freezer, they are warmed to room temperature in approximately thirty-five seconds. This rapid thaw method helps minimize damage to the embryos from ice shards. The embryologist then removes the antifreeze from the embryo and replaces the water lost during freezing. To accomplish this, the embryo is moved through four different solutions over a period of about thirty minutes until all of the cryoprotectant is gone and all of the water is replaced. Once complete, the embryo is warmed to body temperature (98.6°F/37ºC).

You will feel much different after the embryo transfer procedure than you did after the egg retrieval procedure. There may be some mild cramping or spotting from the catheter, but otherwise you should not have any discomfort.

HINT for WOMEN

Wear a panty liner to your embryo transfer in the event you have some mild spotting.

Most clinics have their own recommendations but, in general, you will be asked to lie on your back for thirty minutes or so before being sent home. Another area of controversy deals with the need for bed rest following embryo transfer. More and more studies suggest that bed rest is not required following embryo transfer, so this is a personal decision for you to make. There are instances where your RE may strictly enforce bed rest, but for the most part you need to do what makes you feel most comfortable and what keeps you sane during the two week wait.

Overview of Embryo Transfer

- Pre-implantation genetic diagnosis may be used in order to choose the highest quality embryos for transfer. There is a risk of damage to the developing embryo, so this decision should be made carefully.
- Assisted hatching may be performed to assist the embryo in attaching to the endometrium.
- The timing of the transfer and the number of embryos transferred will vary greatly, with the majority of transfers occurring either on Day 3 or Day 5. Your RE will transfer the least number of embryos possible to give you the best chance at achieving pregnancy.
- The embryo transfer is more relaxed and much less uncomfortable than the egg retrieval, feeling like a Pap smear for most women.
- From the day your embryos come home with you, stay positive, rub your belly and talk to your embies. Like many women, this may be your first real chance of conceiving after many heartaches and years of struggling. Let your embies know that they are loved and fill your body with all those "feel good" endorphins and hormones.
- Make sure to check the status of your remaining embryos to know if you will have any totsicles for future frozen embryo transfer cycles.

Chapter Eleven

Two Week Wait

preparation…suppression…stimulation…egg retrieval…
embryo transfer…two week wait…and beyond

The Agonizing Wait Begins

This portion of your cycle is comprised of the days following embryo transfer to the first scheduled quantitative beta test. The two week wait is used as a general term within the infertility community. It is quite possible that you will not have to wait two weeks, or that you may have to wait longer than two weeks. The waiting period is determined by the day on which you did the transfer, as well your RE's recommendations. Like many couples, you and your partner may find this is the most difficult and stressful portion of an IVF cycle. You will find yourselves going from a very precise regimen of daily calls, updates and injections, to an unregulated time of waiting and thinking. The one medication continued through the two week wait is progesterone.

"I am the master of my fate: I am the captain of my soul."—*William Ernest Henley*

What to Do and Not Do During the Two Week Wait

Much debate surrounds what you should or should not do during the two week wait. For every person or physician who recommends no sex and bed rest, there is another person or physician who states sexual intercourse and normal activity levels are fine. Therefore, your two week wait should be spent as you and your physician feel is best for your individual situation.

Everyone will agree that a low stress situation is best, as is keeping to a healthy lifestyle geared towards impending pregnancy. This means no alcohol, smoking, ibuprofen, caffeine or activities carrying risk of bodily injury, such as heavy lifting, skiing, skydiving, and so on. If you feel in your heart that rest is best, then by all means curl up with a good book or chat online with others during the two week wait. If you would rather keep busy to occupy your mind, use common sense to not overdo it and get the stress relief you need. Remember that it does take time for your ovaries to shrink back to their pre-cycle size, so be aware of this when doing activities.

HINT for WOMEN

Manage your stress with aromatherapy. Aromas thought to aid in stress relief include chamomile, jasmine, lavender, rose and sandalwood.

Implantation Bleeding

You may experience spotting during the two week wait at the time of implantation. This is referred to as implantation bleeding and typically occurs seven to ten days after egg retrieval (for IVFers, egg retrieval corresponds with ovulation). However, it is completely normal to experience *no* spotting during the two week wait. Most likely you will experience some breast tenderness and bloating from the progesterone, hCG trigger shot and/or enlarged ovaries, making it impossible to distinguish between medication-induced symptoms and pregnancy-induced symptoms. Like many women, you may experience cramping similar to an impending period. In fact, you will be certain that Aunt Flo is due to arrive any day with that achy, crampy feeling that normally begins a few days before your period starts. With so many symptoms appearing to signal the arrival of Aunt Flo, you are likely to find yourself under a tremendous amount of stress as you wait for your beta day to arrive.

"We must accept finite disappointment, but we must never lose infinite hope."
—*Martin Luther King, Jr.*

Coping During the Two Week Wait

As previously mentioned, you and your partner will find yourselves going from a very regimented life of injections, ultrasounds and medication changes to an unmonitored period with ample time to think. The daily calls and updates disappear and instead you find yourself counting the days, hours and minutes until your scheduled pregnancy test. And those days seem to last a lifetime. Each day you find yourself scrutinizing every twinge, every cramp, every burp, searching for a sign that you have been successful. Countless trips to the bathroom to check for spotting, hoping for implantation spotting, but praying for nothing at the same time because the spotting could easily be wicked Aunt Flo, there to dash your hopes. Sore breasts one day but not the next; bloating more than usual or some indigestion that comes and goes; mood swings from utter despair because you just know your cycle didn't work; to complete joy that you have a life growing inside you. The insanity of the two week wait gets us all.

HINT for COUPLES

Ask your friends and family to pray for you and keep you in their thoughts. Studies have shown a positive impact from prayer during times of illness and medical treatments.

The absolute best strategy for surviving your two week wait is to stay busy. Occupy your mind and divert your attention elsewhere so that you don't find yourself checking the clock or marking the calendar. Read a book which has absolutely nothing to do with infertility or pregnancy, create scrapbook pages to document the wonderful relationship between you and your loved one, try your hand at a hobby you haven't had time for recently, organize all those photos you have been meaning to get to, or watch funny movies to keep your spirits light.

HINT for WOMEN

Many acupuncturists recommend watching comedies during the two week wait, as they feel laughter can help implantation.

The way to survive the two week wait is to manage your stress and surround yourself with positive energy. You will know what makes you most happy and what brings a smile to your face. Direct your energy into those activities. Pamper yourself—you deserve it. And, as difficult as it may be, try to avoid using home pregnancy tests.

Home Pregnancy Tests

A home pregnancy test (HPT) done prior to the end of the two week wait is *unreliable*. This is important enough to bear repeating: A home pregnancy test done during the two week wait is unreliable! Although you may want to use a HPT to prepare yourselves for beta day, the pain of a negative beta hurts no matter how well you try to prepare. You may hear of IVFers instructed to use a HPT because some clinics have their patients use a home pregnancy test on beta day, asking them to come in for a quantitative beta if the results are positive. This seems to be more of a trend in countries other than the United States.

You may wonder why home pregnancy tests provide no real answers regarding your cycle outcome. The answer lies in the fact that home pregnancy tests are qualitative tests, meaning they give a yes or no answer for the presence of hCG, but do not give a specific value. Human chorionic gonadotropin (hCG) is the hormone produced following implantation, initially by the embryo and later by the placenta. This hormone is found circulating in the blood stream but also spills into your urine, allowing a HPT to check for pregnancy. The earliest you can test with a HPT is seven to ten days post-ovulation (7dpo–10dpo). This is because implantation must occur for hCG to be produced and implantation typically occurs six to twelve days post-ovulation (remember, with an IVF cycle, ovulation corresponds to the day of egg retrieval). When you are assisted with conception, an hCG trigger shot is used to induce final maturation of developing eggs before egg retrieval, and you may receive an additional hCG injection during your treatment to aid in adequate progesterone production by the uterus. Home pregnancy tests do not distinguish between hCG produced from the placenta or injected hCG. Therefore, when you receive an hCG trigger shot, you must wait seven to fourteen days from the hCG injection before testing with a home pregnancy test to ensure the injected hCG is out of your system. If you receive a larger hCG injection dose, you should wait at least fourteen days. If you receive a smaller hCG injection dose, you may have it out of your system as early as seven days. If you do not wait for the injected hCG to clear your system, there is no way of knowing if the HPT is detecting placental hCG or injected hCG.

No test is 100 percent accurate and other factors contribute to the reliability of the test. First morning urine is best so that the hCG level is not diluted. One of the key limiting factors of a home pregnancy test is its sensitivity, meaning the lowest level of hCG it can detect. This sensitivity can vary greatly among the numerous brands of home pregnancy tests on the market. Presence of blood or protein in the urine can cause an inaccurate test reading, as can certain drugs. There are five possible outcomes when testing with a HPT: (1) invalid test, (2) true positive, (3) false positive, (4) true negative, (4) false negative.

An invalid test occurs when the control window does not appear as a positive. No matter what the test reads, if the control window does not appear as a positive, the entire test is useless. A positive result can be either a true positive, meaning you are pregnant, or a false positive, meaning the test is detecting hCG from an injection, or the hCG detected is not from a viable pregnancy, such as a chemical pregnancy. A negative result can be either a true negative, meaning you are not pregnant, or a false negative, indicating the hCG level is below that particular brand's sensitivity but you are, actually, pregnant.

Keep in mind that false negatives do occur, especially when testing too early. If you begin testing too early, you can get a false positive from the hCG trigger remaining in your system, or get a false negative because your levels are not high enough to be detected yet. In the case of late implantation, a false negative HPT can even occur on the day of the scheduled beta. It is also important to realize that the presence of hCG does not translate to a viable pregnancy. As you can see, home pregnancy tests have earned the name of "evil pee stick" for a reason among IVFers. You and your partner need to make your own decision about whether to test with a home pregnancy test. Just bear in mind that the only result that can be completely trusted is a quantitative beta hCG blood test performed by your physician or lab.

The Beta

Your entire journey to this point has been riddled with ups and downs, joys and worries, and more needle sticks than you ever thought possible. And it all comes down to this all-important needle stick at the end of your two week wait—the beta hCG test, or "the beta," as IVFers call it. This test is different from testing with a home pregnancy test because it is a quantitative test that assigns an actual numeric value for the level of hCG detected in the blood. There is no worry of a diluted sample and a very small amount of hCG can be detected. Again, there are variations among labs and clinics as to what constitutes a positive beta. This is mainly due to the variation in the time between embryo transfer and actual testing, with some clinics waiting less than two weeks and some waiting longer. Always check with your clinic to make sure you understand what qualifies as a positive beta with your clinic's laboratory.

Having a good support network is crucial during and after the two week wait. During the wait, you may fear the worst, as you have ample time to contemplate the odds facing you. Oftentimes you will go back over your cycle, finding fault and areas where you feel you could have done better to improve your chances of pregnancy. The outcome of the two week wait is left to the strength and determination of the transferred embryos, so it is important to stay positive and look to the future.

HINT for GUYS

Be positive and encourage your loved one during the two week wait. Don't be judgmental about her worries or anxieties, and remind her just how far you *have* come.

There is only a limited window of uterine receptivity (even with unassisted conception the window lasts only a few days). This means there is only a short time period in which the uterus is receptive to the embryo and there is only a short time period during which the embryo can actually implant. You have done a great job getting to this point. Now it is out of your hands and you must wait. No matter what symptoms you may or may not be having, always have your beta test. It is very common for women to experience bleeding in early pregnancy, so even if you are actively bleeding you need to have your beta drawn. If you have succumbed to the evil pee stick and get a negative test, have your beta regardless. Women have had a negative HPT on the day of their beta and been pregnant with a healthy little one. Don't leave anything to chance; don't give up hope until your beta results arrive.

A Negative Beta Test

Make sure you have privacy when you get the call from your clinic and have a support person close by for good or bad news. A negative beta is a crushing disappointment, not a failure. You did an amazing job making it as far as the two week wait, and no matter how deeply you hurt, don't feel a negative cycle is a personal failure.

HINT for COUPLES

Decide in advance who will receive the results of your beta test. If at all possible, take the call at home rather than at work. Even if you feel you have prepared yourself by using a HPT, actually hearing the words, "Your beta is negative. You are not pregnant," can be quite difficult and can bring on some very intense emotions.

A Positive Beta Test

If you are blessed with a positive beta, remember that the rise in your beta numbers over the next few days will be a better predictor of a viable pregnancy than any single number. Celebrate this milestone and stay positive as you again find yourself counting the days. At the end of the two week wait, the waiting continues for some while the healing begins for others.

Overview of the Two Week Wait

- The waiting period between transfer day and the beta is the most stressful portion of an in vitro cycle, so it is important to find ways to occupy your mind and stay positive.

- Avoid using a home pregnancy test since the results really don't have the same value as a quantitative test. Remember, you are testing much earlier than the general population and much can happen in the early days and weeks following transfer.

- Do not be upset if you don't have implantation spotting. Many women will not experience this and go on to have healthy pregnancies.

- ALWAYS have your beta test, even if you are convinced your cycle did not work. Many women have been pleasantly surprised on beta day when they thought all was lost.

Chapter Twelve

And Beyond

*preparation…suppression…stimulation…egg retrieval…
embryo transfer…two week wait…and beyond*

The Journey Beyond the Beta

Although you may consider your cycle finished once you receive your beta results, I believe the weeks following the beta really are the closing weeks of an in vitro cycle. The two week wait culminates with a simple blood test that may bring intense sadness, incredible joy or confusion. The first few weeks beyond the two week wait can still be quite the roller coaster ride for you and your partner—those weeks are often emotionally charged and require even better coping skills.

"Have you come to the Red Sea place in your life?
Where, in spite of all you can do, there is no way
out, there is no way back, there is no other way but
through."—*Annie Johnson Flint*

The Emotions of a Negative Beta

News of a negative beta can be crushing. Sadness and anger can frequently overcome you, especially in the case of a "perfect cycle." Intense swings in mood happen easily, as hormones have still not returned to normal levels. No matter what has been done to prepare for a negative beta, your heart can't help but break after cheering your embies on and lovingly bringing them home.

Failure to Implant

One area that remains a stumbling block to achieving success with an in vitro cycle is failure of the embryo to implant. With regards to uterine receptivity, the cells lining the uterus undergo specific changes which make the uterus highly receptive to the implanting embryo. This period of maximum sensitivity is called the receptive phase. During the receptive phase the embryo can implant, but outside this receptive phase, the uterus will resist attachment of the blastocyst.[19]

Reasons Your Embryos May Have Failed to Implant

- Genetic abnormalities
- Abnormal embryo development due to the process of IVF, be it the lab setting, timing of transfer or shock of transfer
- Abnormally thick shell preventing the embryo from hatching
- Unreceptive uterus
- Immune factors
- Unknown reasons

Coping with a negative beta is a grieving process for you and it takes time to work through the barrage of emotions a negative test brings. Many times, cycle buddies will receive good news and it is easy to feel left out and punished. Despair and sadness make trying another cycle seem impossible, emotionally and physically. You never go into a cycle feeling you will add to the disheartening failure statistics. The hope you once clung onto to get you through the tough days simply vanishes with a single phone call.

How Men Cope Differently

What can make matters worse is that your partner, similar to many men, will likely react to news of a failed cycle with what seems a cold, problem-solving attitude: "We'll get pregnant next time." You, however, will likely react with a sense of doom. "The obstacles are too great. If everything went right with this cycle, and we still got a negative, how can another cycle be any different?" It is very easy for you and your partner to drift apart because you are in a vulnerable, emotional state and may feel anger that your partner is not experiencing the same degree of pain.

In some cases, your partner may not have become as attached to the transferred embryos. Often, his pain is quite deep but he works to hide it, wishing to be the strong one in the relationship and not really having an avenue for venting the overwhelming emotions he is feeling. It is important to remember that we each have our own way of dealing with difficult events in our life, but through it all the lines of communication need to remain open and honest after receiving a negative beta. You took on this challenge together as a team and this aspect of your cycle should also be tackled as a team. Together, you are much stronger than you think!

> "And the day came when the risk it took to remain tight inside the bud was more painful than the risk it took to blossom."—*Anaïs Nin*

Taking Time to Heal

It is very tempting to begin another cycle immediately. You may feel you have a momentum going, or feel becoming pregnant will ease the pain of failing with your previous cycle. Although these are both legitimate reasons to forge forward, it is prudent to allow yourselves the opportunity to truly deal with a failed cycle. Not only has your mind been through a tremendously stressful undertaking, but your body has gone through significant hormonal changes and procedures. Many women find they gain on average seven to twelve pounds with their in vitro cycle from the stress, enlarged ovaries and fluid retention. Never underestimate what you have accomplished, even in the event of a negative beta. You have pushed your body to limits it has never been asked to reach before, you have subjected yourself to medications and monitoring, you have bottomed out your hormones and then quickly built them beyond their normal levels, and you have sacrificed and compromised to be given the chance at conceiving a child of your own. Any one of these is monumental in and of itself, and you have done them all in a matter of weeks.

Time is always the enemy when battling infertility, but give yourselves the time you need and deserve to recover from the journey you have taken before placing your feet back on the path again. It is important to be healthy in mind, body and spirit when cycling, and that doesn't happen in a day or two. Each cycle brings us closer to our dreams and gives us more insight to our individual obstacles. Learn from a failed cycle, adapt from a failed cycle, and never lose sight of what brought you to the doorstep of your RE. A baby is a wonderful dream to chase. Whether you trip, stumble or even fall flat on your face, in the end the reward washes away the pain and the disappointment gathered along the way.

The Emotions of a Positive Beta

If you are lucky enough to receive news of a positive beta, you must begin the dreaded numbers game. A game none of us wish to play, but find ourselves drawn into against our will. You likely dreamt of the day your positive beta would arrive, thinking it would be the most glorious day and the end to your worries and struggles. Yet, more often than not, it is the beginning of an entirely different struggle—the struggle to go to term with your pregnancy. Although, like many couples, you may believe the first beta is a tell-all test, it is but the first step towards determining if your pregnancy is a viable one.

Understanding Rising Betas

Most clinics will perform two to three beta tests spread out over two to three-day intervals to watch for a trend in the rise of beta numbers. A single beta number does not predict the viability of a pregnancy; low betas often lead to healthy babies and high betas often lead to miscarriage. It is the sad fact we all must face when we make it to this stage of the baby chase. Most often, the beta number should at minimum double every two to three days (48-72 hours) during the first four weeks of gestation. Since there can be wide variation in beta numbers, your physician is watching for a trend of increasing levels. If a beta number does not double over a two to three day period, it does NOT doom the pregnancy. Physicians work by a theory that the largest portion of the population will fall within the guidelines set forth, but not everyone follows the average of the population. As I always tell my support group members, "Sometimes the embryos don't read the book."

It is also important to remember that you will test much earlier than those conceiving without medical assistance, which puts you in the unique position of monitoring changes in beta numbers other couples are oblivious to by time they are seen by an obstetrician.

Many times, more than one embryo will implant but not all implanted embryos will survive, commonly referred to as "vanishing twin syndrome" among the infertile population. This can occur at any time and can alter the expected rise in beta numbers. Should multiple embryos implant and give an initial high beta, when one or more of the embryos halts in development, the beta levels may continue to rise, but not at the rate of doubling every two to three days, even though you can go on to carry a healthy pregnancy to term. As the pregnancy progresses, the time it takes for beta numbers to double will lengthen until hCG levels reach their peak around eight to eleven weeks gestation, at which time levels decline somewhat before leveling off for the remainder of the pregnancy.

Each passing stage brings greater confidence in a viable pregnancy, but, unfortunately, not even fantastic beta numbers guarantee success after in vitro fertilization. The early ultrasounds following your betas will be much stronger predictors; so, again, you find yourself counting the weeks, hoping for progression with each ultrasound. Because your physician is monitoring your pregnancy at such an early stage, it is necessary to perform ultrasound evaluations with a vaginal probe, the same as when she monitored your follicles during your cycle. This is because transabdominal ultrasound cannot adequately visualize the tiny structures which mark the earliest development of a pregnancy.

Ectopic Pregnancy

An ectopic pregnancy is a risk of in vitro fertilization and occurs at the rate of 4.5 percent, more than double the 2 percent rate of the general population.[20] Your doctor can make the diagnosis of an ectopic pregnancy when the beta levels do not rise as expected and when she is unable to find an embryo within the uterus or finds the embryo within the Fallopian tube (the most common site of an ectopic pregnancy). There are risk factors for ectopic pregnancy specific to assisted reproductive technologies, including the type of ART, cause of infertility, and number of embryos transferred. Couples using zygote intrafallopian transfer (ZIFT) are twice as likely to experience an ectopic pregnancy, as are couples with the diagnosis of tubal factor infertility. Couples who transfer three or more embryos are also at increased risk for an ectopic pregnancy.[21]

Early Ultrasound in Pregnancy

When pregnancy occurs within the uterus, the earliest visible gestational sac is seen at four and one-half weeks (almost all should be seen by five weeks), and is quite small, measuring only about 2 mm in diameter. The first landmark identifying a *true* gestational sac is the yolk sac, which is usually seen around five to six weeks. The yolk sac appears as a spherical membrane and is readily seen when the gestational sac measures 8 to10 mm. At minimum, the gestational sac should be visible on average when the hCG levels are between 1,000 to 2,000 mIU/ml, but ranges as great as 629-2,188 mIU/ml have been reported (mIU/ml is the unit of measurement used when measuring hCG levels).[22]

The embryo will appear around five and a half to six weeks gestation and is seen as a thickening on the margin of the yolk sac. The heartbeat, seen as a flutter within the embryo, is first evident just after six weeks but may not be visible until seven weeks gestation. It is possible for a small, normal embryo to not have a heartbeat just after six weeks, but to have a heartbeat on a follow-up ultrasound, five to seven days later.[23]

Blighted Ovum/Chemical Pregnancy

After the excitement of a positive beta, your dreams may be shattered when ultrasound reveals either a blighted ovum (chemical pregnancy) or no heartbeat. A blighted ovum is technically termed anembryonic gestation. In this instance, a gestational sac forms without the subsequent development of an embryo. Most likely this is due to early embryonic death and the result is a gestational sac that remains empty with no distinguishable structures within it. Although gestational sacs up to 20 mm not showing an embryo may continue as a normal pregnancy, usually a gestational sac greater than 18 mm in diameter without an embryo is considered abnormal and is not likely to progress.[24] Failure to develop a heartbeat is also often due to early embryonic death. As infertility patients, we must deal with these heartaches that couples who conceive unassisted are unaware of, as many of those pregnancies would go largely undetected.

Presence of a heartbeat on ultrasound is very reassuring and is associated with approximately a 70 percent continuance rate.[25] You will often hear that early miscarriage plagues many in vitro couples, but typically the rates are similar to those experienced by couples conceiving without medical assistance, approximately 15 to 20 percent of recognized pregnancies.[26] IVFers often seem to have higher rates of miscarriage due to early testing and other factors such as advanced maternal age and multiple gestations. As a pregnancy progresses, the prognosis of carrying a healthy baby to term improves.

During the early weeks of pregnancy, take good care of yourself. Stick to a healthy lifestyle and follow your doctor's orders. All you can do is provide the healthiest and safest environment possible for your little one(s); the rest is left to Mother Nature and the will and strength of your baby. Enjoy every moment to the fullest and remain positive that your dream really has come true!

Overview of And Beyond

- The days and weeks following your beta really are part of your in vitro cycle and need to be traversed with understanding and acceptance of your cycle outcome.

- Express your emotions should you receive a negative beta. Face the deep, ugly feelings and vent them to your fertility friends and partner. It is okay to be angry. It is okay to be sad. It is okay to feel all is lost. This is part of the grieving process. In time, you will find acceptance and seek answers. Most often your RE will not have any answer for why your cycle failed, but know that a failed cycle does not mean your next cycle will suffer the same fate. Conception through IVF is a battle of statistics, just as it is with couples attempting to conceive without medical assistance. So many couples become parents with subsequent cycles, be it fresh cycles or frozen ones. Only you know to what lengths you can stretch in chasing your dream. Give yourself time to heal and regain your strength, then forge forward with a positive attitude and the knowledge you need to find success.

- Should you find success with your cycle, celebrate. This is no small feat you have just accomplished. Have compassion when sharing your updates—many of your friends may still be struggling. Don't shut yourself off from your friends still trying to conceive, but let them approach you with questions about your pregnancy rather than offering updates. Having reached such a monumental milestone, your encouragement can help them find strength for their own efforts. Try to enjoy your time as a mother-to-be. Loss is heartbreaking, whether it happens in the first few weeks, or later in your pregnancy. There are no guarantees and the fear never really goes away, even after delivery. But there is no greater joy than becoming a mother. Motherhood should be celebrated as the incredible blessing it is.

Chapter Thirteen

Factors Affecting IVF Cycle Outcome

Many couples attempting to conceive with the help of assisted reproductive technologies such as in vitro fertilization and frozen embryo transfer find themselves feeling helpless during their cycle. For the most part, couples must hand control over to their reproductive endocrinologist, often someone they just met within the past few weeks. Not only are all medication dosages timed and regulated, ultrasound evaluations and even sexual intercourse are placed on a timetable beyond the couple's control. Some factors, such as age, ethnic background, and medical diagnoses are beyond anyone's control, but couples can devote themselves to certain lifestyle changes to improve their chances of becoming pregnant. It is also worthwhile for couples to educate themselves about the specific obstacles they may face so that their expectations are in line with their cycle. Although there is not always conclusive evidence to back these recommendations, all couples can benefit from a healthy approach to cycling. Undergoing in vitro is not a way to sidestep these lifestyle changes! These factors can directly affect the chances of pregnancy and of having a successful IVF cycle.

Factors known to influence the chances of conception with ART include, but are not limited to, the following: caffeine, alcohol, recreational drugs, weight, vitamins and supplements, medications, stress, smoking, age, ovarian cysts, polycystic ovarian syndrome, thyroid disease, endometriosis, decreased ovarian reserve, autoimmune factors, male factor requiring ICSI, hydrosalpinx, race, type of ovarian stimulation, junctional zone changes, timing of hCG trigger, interval between hCG trigger and egg retrieval, and ovarian hyperstimulation syndrome.

Caffeine

Caffeine is thought to interfere with fertility in both men (decreased sperm motility) and women. This is one area where each physician may have her own recommendations. The American Pregnancy Association recommends consuming less than 300 mg of caffeine a day; greater than 300 mg/day may reduce fertility as much as 27 percent.[27] Many physicians will recommend limiting coffee intake to one to two cups a day, or limiting soda intake to one or two 12 ounce cans a day. Dr. Alice Domar, Ph.D., recommends you consume less than 59 mg of caffeine a day to improve success following in vitro fertilization.[28]

Coffee is a very common form of caffeine consumption for couples, but both the type of coffee bean and the preparation method greatly affect the caffeine content of coffee. Specialty coffee blends (such as espresso) often have much higher caffeine content. It is also important to remember that many prescription and over-the-counter medications such as diuretics, cold formulas and pain relievers, contain caffeine. Caffeine content should be available on product labeling, and it is always a good idea to check this to avoid excessive caffeine intake.

Some general caffeine contents:
- Milk chocolate (1 oz.)—3-6 mg
- Dark chocolate (1 oz.)—20-25 mg
- Coca-Cola (12 fl. oz. can)—34 mg
- Pepsi (12 fl. oz. can)—38 mg
- Brewed coffee (8 fl. oz.)—40-180 mg
- Instant coffee (8 fl. oz.)—30-120 mg

Alcohol

Both acute (one-time consumption) and chronic alcohol consumption have been associated with decreased levels of testosterone in men.[29] Alcohol also affects sperm and can cause a decreased percentage of normal sperm morphology, count and motility.[30] Some physicians will recommend abstinence from alcohol during a cycle or limiting intake to two ounces or less twice a week.[31] Since alcohol is known to be very detrimental to a developing fetus, the safest lifestyle for the woman is to also avoid alcohol in the event her cycle is indeed a success.

Recreational Drugs

Drugs such as heroin, cocaine, marijuana, and anabolic steroids all have detrimental effects on the reproductive system. Heroin use can lead to decreased LH and testosterone levels in men, as well as decreased sperm count, decreased sperm motility and increased abnormal morphology in sperm.[32] Heroin use in women can significantly disrupt the normal menstrual cycle through its effects on LH and FSH. Cocaine leads to decreased sperm count and motility, and leads to increased abnormal sperm morphology. Marijuana use may lower testosterone levels and decrease sperm quality (lowered sperm count and motility with increased abnormal morphology). Marijuana remains in the testes for more than two weeks, so even occasional use can be detrimental.[33] Anabolic steroids lead to decreased testosterone and decreased sperm count.

Weight

Although the media tends to address the issue of obesity more prominently, men and women falling below their ideal body weight have poorer pregnancy outcomes as well as those battling the bulge. It is important to maintain a healthy weight as determined by one's age and height to improve the chances of success with ART. With obesity, even a slight reduction in body fat can improve the chances of conception following an IVF cycle. Overweight and obese women tend to be resistant to stimulation medications, requiring higher doses. Obese women will often have displaced ovaries, making it more difficult to reach them during egg retrieval. Increased body fat can also make ultrasound imaging more difficult. The American Society for Reproductive Medicine outlines the fertility issues for obese women as being at increased risk during fertility surgery, being at increased risk for miscarriage, and having lower success rates with fertility treatments. Weight loss of as little as 5 to 10 percent may dramatically improve pregnancy rates in obese women.[34]

Women significantly below their ideal weight often experience a shutdown of their reproductive system as a mechanism of preventing pregnancy and may run the risk of other serious issues if they are malnourished before embarking on an in vitro cycle.

Like women, men who are below or above their ideal body weight may face fertility issues. One study demonstrated that men with a low body mass index (BMI, defined as less than 20 kg/m_2) may have a 36 percent lower sperm count and a 28 percent reduction in sperm concentration compared to men with a normal BMI. Interestingly, obese men also demonstrate changes in their sperm. Men with a high BMI (defined as greater than 25 kg/m_2) may have a 24 percent lower sperm count and a 22 percent reduction in sperm concentration compared to men with a normal BMI. As a man's body mass index increases, his testosterone levels decrease.[35]

Vitamins and Supplements

Much discussion on improving health revolves around free radicals and their effect on the human body and immune system. Free radicals can attack and destroy the delicate membrane that surrounds the sperm, impairing conception. Infertile men have a higher concentration of free radicals in their semen compared to fertile men and therefore may benefit from vitamins and other antioxidants. Consider the following vitamins based on a physician's recommendations:

- Zinc may be beneficial in men with low testosterone levels, as zinc increases testosterone levels and improves sperm production. One of the best natural sources for zinc is oysters.
- Vitamin C has antioxidant properties as well as acts to reduce sperm agglutination (a condition where the sperm stick to each other, impeding fertility). Vitamin C can improve sperm quality in smokers.
- Vitamin E has antioxidant properties.

- Selenium can increase sperm motility.[36]
- Lycopene has antioxidant properties.[37]

Wheat grass, flaxseed oil and DHA oils may lower FSH in women with elevated levels. It is currently believed that at least two ounces of wheatgrass per day may be of benefit. Flaxseed oil, as well as DHA, may reduce an elevated FSH level. However, not all omega-3 oils are the same. A number of studies show a range of benefits from fish oil, especially from the EPA and DHA fatty acids. Other oils, like flaxseed oil, have less evidence of benefits compared to fish oil. Flaxseed oil primarily contains the omega-3 fatty acid called alpha-linolenic acid, some of which is partly converted to EPA by the body. The EPA from flaxseed oil can have some of the same benefits as fish oil and is a good alternative for those unable to stomach the taste of the fish oils.[38]

When discussing the use of supplements, there are conflicting reports on the safety and benefits of some supplements. Therefore, many reproductive endocrinologists prefer their patients refrain from using supplements during their cycle as their effect on a controlled hyperstimulation cycle is vastly unknown. Even vitamins taken in excessive doses can be detrimental to your health, so please, always consult with your doctor before taking any supplements.

Medications

As mentioned previously, some diuretics, cold formulas and pain relievers contain caffeine and should be avoided. Cimetidine decreases testosterone levels and may affect sperm production.[39] Other medications that may have a negative impact on sperm quality include calcium channel blockers (taken for elevated blood pressure), sulfasalazine and mercaptopurine (taken for Crohn's disease), colchicine and allopurinol (taken for gout), and cyclosporine (taken after organ transplant).[40] It is important for the woman to avoid using nonsteroidal, anti-inflammatory medications such as ibuprofen, as these medications block progesterone.

If you are unsure whether your current medications may negatively impact your cycle, consult with your clinic to get their specific recommendations.

Stress

Stress may be the one factor a couple will find almost impossible to control during a cycle. The process of in vitro itself is very taxing, making a certain level of stress unavoidable. One study examined the effects of stress on cycling and found women who are concerned about their procedure may have as much as 20 percent fewer eggs retrieved and 19 percent fewer eggs fertilized compared to women who worry less about their cycle. The study also found that women who are very concerned over missing work may have as much as 30 percent fewer eggs fertilized.[41] Baseline acute and chronic stress affects the number of oocytes retrieved and fertilization rates, and also impacts pregnancy and live births. Interestingly, stress related to the process of in vitro itself only affects the number of oocytes retrieved and fertilization rates.[42] Stress in men leads to decreased sperm count, volume and concentration due to decreased LH and testosterone production.[43]

Smoking

Cigarette smoke, both firsthand and secondhand, significantly affects both the man's fertility and the woman's fertility. Even more alarming is recent research revolving around the effects of secondhand smoke inhalation as either sidestream smoke (smoke inhaled from a burning cigarette), or passive smoke (exhaled by the smoker), where a nicotine metabolite has been found in the follicular fluid of nonsmoking couples. The degree of damage done by smoking is dependent on the amount smoked and the length of time the individual has smoked. Regular smoking decreases the size and movement of sperm and, to a lesser extent, negatively impacts their morphology. Smoking also lowers a man's sperm count.

Smoking cigarettes significantly affects a woman's reproductive health as well. Compared to women who do not smoke, women who smoke have poorer quality eggs and embryos.[44] The ASRM impresses upon women that compared to nonsmokers, smokers have decreased ovarian reserves and have ovaries that are less responsive to stimulation medications used during a cycle. Smokers have fewer oocytes (eggs) retrieved and fertilized compared to nonsmokers and also suffer from lower pregnancy rates when compared to nonsmokers.

One study found a nine percent risk of a failed IVF or gamete intrafallopian transfer (GIFT) cycle for each year a woman smokes, and smokers may require twice the number of attempts at IVF or GIFT to find success in comparison to nonsmokers.[45] Nicotine and other chemicals present in cigarettes interfere with the production of estrogen and cause the woman's eggs to be more prone to genetic abnormalities, according to the ASRM. Smokers often require higher doses of stimulation medications.[46] Smoking also appears to accelerate atresia of oocytes, leading to early menopause. Although smoking will cause long-term damage to the ovaries (smoking decreases a woman's ovarian reserve), some physicians feel the effects of smoking on current fertility may no longer be a factor three to four months after quitting.[47]

Age

A woman's age is more of a limiting factor for achieving pregnancy than the age of the man. Although men do experience a natural decrease in testosterone levels and have a decrease in normal sperm morphology and motility as they age, no maximum age has been determined at which a man can no longer father a child. Unfortunately, this is not true for women. In fact, the ASRM feels that a woman's age is the most important predictor of her potential to become pregnant when utilizing her own eggs (donor eggs from a younger egg donor show increased success rates, providing evidence that the egg and embryo quality is a significant limiting factor).

As a woman ages, her quantity and quality of eggs decrease steadily until her ovaries shut down completely at menopause. Because a woman is born with all the eggs she will ever have (in contrast to men who continue to produce sperm throughout their life), as her age increases she has fewer and fewer eggs available and they are of poorer quality. Older eggs demonstrate a higher incidence of genetic abnormalities, which may not lower fertilization rates but lower pregnancy rates. As a woman ages, her ovaries become less responsive to gonadotropins and oftentimes older women produce fewer follicles and oocytes in spite of the higher doses of stimulation medications. When utilizing intracytoplasmic sperm injection during an in vitro cycle, increased maternal age does not impact fertilization rates but does lower pregnancy rates.[48]

The pregnancy rates following a cycle utilizing controlled hyperstimulation with gonadotropins in women older than forty years of age is a disheartening 5 to 8 percent per treatment according to the ASRM.[49] This is due to several factors including a decrease in embryo development following fertilization, a decrease in embryo implantation rates and an increase in miscarriage rates.

Ovarian Cysts

Although women may have preexisting ovarian cysts, cysts can develop during an in vitro fertilization cycle due to medications. There is conflicting and confusing data regarding the effect of ovarian cysts on IVF outcome as well as the management of them, as each physician has her own set of recommendations. Studies on ovarian cysts that develop during an in vitro cycle, show that cysts have a negative impact on cycle outcome if they are functional as determined by elevated estradiol levels. Functional cysts occur in at least five percent of cycles with GnRHa use and occur more frequently if the serum progesterone level is low when beginning the GnRHa.[50] Cysts may also negatively affect success if they become large enough to jeopardize the ovarian blood supply or cause torsion of the ovary. However, it is possible for a woman to find success following an in vitro cycle in the presence of an ovarian cyst.

Polycystic Ovarian Syndrome

Women with polycystic ovarian syndrome will have elevated testosterone levels as well as elevated LH and FSH levels. An elevated FSH level is associated with poorer quality eggs and embryos.[51] Elevated testosterone levels can down regulate estrogen receptors within the uterine lining, thereby diminishing the potential for implantation.

Thyroid Disease

Women living with thyroid disease will have elevated LH and FSH levels, and thus poorer quality eggs and embryos. This condition may progress to a condition called primary ovarian failure where proteins and white blood cells in the blood attack proteins in the ovaries, leading to premature menopause. Antithyroid antibodies (antithyroglobulin antibodies (ATA) and antimicrosomal antibodies (AMA) are associated with two times higher rate of miscarriage and implantation failure, and are independent markers for pregnancies at risk for miscarriage.[52] Since sperm development is closely tied to normal thyroid hormone levels, hypo- and hyperthyroidism can affect sperm production.[53]

Endometriosis

Women suffering from endometriosis will have poorer quality embryos.[54]

Decreased Ovarian Reserve

Decreased ovarian reserve provides a greater challenge to achieving pregnancy as it is often the main infertility issue facing women of advanced age. This condition does occur in younger women as well and is often called early menopause. Decreased ovarian reserve is diagnosed by testing FSH and/or E2 levels, as well as LH levels on specific days of the woman's menstrual cycle. Ovarian reserve is further evaluated by the antral follicle count and ovarian volume. An elevated FSH or E2 level on Day 3 of a woman's cycle is associated with lower pregnancy rates with in vitro fertilization. Newer research has also shown that women with an elevated LH level on Day 3 have a poor pregnancy outcome with assisted reproductive technologies. An elevated FSH level on cycle Day 3 or Day 10 during a clomiphene citrate challenge test also predicts a lower pregnancy rate with ART.[55] An antral follicle count of less than five indicates decreased ovarian reserve and is often associated with a significantly decreased pregnancy rate.[56]

Autoimmune Issues

There are numerous autoimmune conditions that may impact a couple's fertility. Elevated LH levels are seen with some autoimmune disorders. Sperm antibodies are abnormal proteins that attack sperm, causing impaired movement or clumping. These antibodies are produced by women and also by men, with the man's antibodies attacking his own sperm. Natural killer cells are lymphocytes that function during the normal cycle of a woman. Studies show that in some women, these natural killer cells are at increased activity levels and contribute or lead to failure to implant.[57] Antiphospholipid antibodies (APA) are nonspecific autoantibodies frequently associated with endometriosis and pelvic adhesions.[58]

Male Factor Requiring ICSI

Lack of sperm motility causes the greatest negative impact on fertilization and pregnancy rates.[59]

Hydrosalpinx

The presence of fluid in the Fallopian tubes (known as hydrosalpinx) has been shown to lower the success rates of in vitro fertilization due to decreased rates of implantation. The lowered implantation rate is thought to be due to either a direct toxic effect of the fluid on the developing embryo or a negative impact on the uterine receptivity. Pregnancy rates may be as much as 50 percent lower with hydrosalpinx and miscarriage rates may be as much as two times higher with hydrosalpinx.[60]

Race

In a study that focused on IVF and race, it was noted that black and Asian women may have a lower overall birth rate compared to white and Hispanic women. Black women are also more likely to have a miscarriage when they become pregnant. The differences in race are only apparent with fresh in vitro cycles. No difference was noted with frozen embryo transfers.[61]

Type of Ovarian Stimulation

Although there is conflicting evidence regarding the best protocol for an IVF cycle, recent studies point to no difference in outcomes in cycles that include down regulation (suppression). However, in cycles *without* down regulation using rhFSH (does not contain LH), women seem to produce better quality eggs and embryos when compared to cycles using HMG.[62]

Junctional Zone Changes

The junctional zone is the inner most layer of the myometrium (muscle layer of the uterus). This area impacts uterine receptivity and embryo implantation. A pronounced change in the junctional zone (thinner at Day 8 and then significantly thicker at embryo transfer) seems to be associated with better IVF success.[63]

Timing of hCG Trigger Shot

This timing directly affects the egg and embryo quality, making it important for patients to follow their RE's instructions closely.[64]

Interval Between hCG Trigger and ER

As with the timing of the trigger shot, the interval between the trigger and retrieval is precisely timed and deviation from this can impair both the egg and embryo quality.[65]

Ovarian Hyperstimulation Syndrome

Ovarian hyperstimulation syndrome (OHSS) is distinguished as either early or late. Early OHSS relates to an excessive pre-ovulatory response to stimulation, while late OHSS occurs with pregnancy (late OHSS does not appear to be related to early OHSS).[66] Late OHSS is not covered in this section because it occurs following conception. In early OHSS, a significantly higher number of eggs are retrieved compared to cycles where OHSS does not develop. With similar fertilization rates, women with OHSS tend to have a significantly higher number of viable embryos. However, implantation and pregnancy rates appear to be similar between OHSS and non-OHSS cycles[67] (data and opinions vary on this point, with some RE's feeling that women who experience OHSS tend to have better quality embryos and therefore slightly higher pregnancy rates). There is also conflicting data regarding oocyte quality in instances of severe OHSS. Some studies indicate no decrease in the quality of eggs with severe OHSS, while other opinions reflect decreased oocyte quality and pregnancy rates in cases of severe OHSS. These differences may become sorted out as more studies compare egg quality and pregnancy rates based on the level of estrogen.

Although many factors play a role in achieving a positive beta, many of them are beyond a couple's control. A couple's physical health, mindset, and cycle protocol as well as the people enlisted to help the couple conceive, all influence the outcome of a cycle. Each couple must be realistic when deciding to go the route of in vitro fertilization. It has been a wonderful option for so many couples and continues to evolve as a technical procedure. In vitro fertilization is a beacon of hope that every couple should consider moving towards, regardless if the statistics look grim. Your cycle could very well contribute to the success rates and bring you a beautiful baby to cherish for a lifetime.

Chapter Fourteen

The Beauty of Alphabet Blessings

When Jeff and I became parents, we didn't lose our title as an infertile couple, but we did graduate to become infertility survivors. In the first minute of his life, my son Nicholas accomplished what I couldn't accomplish in five years. He healed the wounds and scars placed on my heart and soul by our

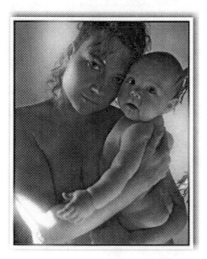

first lost pregnancy and our years of trying to conceive. I gazed at our child, a true blessing, a gift to be loved and cherished for all our lives. The terrible physical and emotional pain I had dealt with to reach that moment in time paled next to his beauty and pureness of soul. The first few weeks home with Nicholas were some of the most intensely emotional days of my life. I couldn't stop gazing at him or touching him. It seemed as though he was all that was good, wrapped up in a tiny little bundle and bestowed upon me, a true gift after so many years of feeling punished.

These first years have been more demanding and more fun than I ever imagined possible. The incredible joy of watching Nicholas and Jeff together, whether running through the house, splashing in the tub or snuggling on the couch, dulls the memories of many tear-filled nights. The pride of seeing my parents interact with Nicholas tightens my chest, knowing they may never have had the chance if it weren't for in vitro fertilization. The happiness of hearing Nicholas roll with laughter as my sister and nephew tickle him fills me with such contentment. The smiles that light up the faces of Jeff's parents warm my heart beyond words. The incredible love I feel for my son is overpowering and intoxicating.

In vitro fertilization has given Jeff and me a chance; not just a chance to become pregnant, but a chance to build a family that extends beyond the walls of our home. We now have the opportunity to experience life as parents and, we hope, one day as grandparents. My sister has been given the chance to know life as Auntie and her son is able to know the joy of hanging out with his cousin. One day our parents may be given the title of great-grandparents. Having Nicholas has given us all the chance to experience life as we hadn't before, to step into a new realm of family, and to connect our hearts through our love for the amazing little boy in vitro blessed us with.

When you find so much happiness and love through assisted conception, it changes how you view life. You come to understand the value of even the tiniest aspects of life and you find yourself unwilling to accept the harshness of others who are oblivious to what it really means to cycle in order to have a child. Before our cycle, I never thought twice about the words test tube baby, but now it turns my stomach to hear those words. It removes the very human aspect of assisted conception: a struggle of two loving individuals willing to sacrifice so much in order to create life. No one refers to babies born via cesarean section as Pfannenstiel babies, yet this is the mechanism of their birth. Medicine aids many couples at different points along their own path to parenthood. IVFers simply have their assistance at the very start of their journey and should never be made to feel that their undertaking is wrong, unethical or unnecessary. By reading this book, I hope you walk away with the sense that in vitro is a very human experience and that the children born of IVF are beautiful blessings and gifts—anything but test tube babies.

I also hope that after reading this book you will see conception for the fertile population as unassisted rather than natural. To refer to natural conception somehow imparts the sense that IVF is unnatural, and although there are religious doctrines making such claims, conception for an IVF couple is driven by love and determination and is just as pure as unassisted conception. Every IVF couple should feel immense pride for their triumph over the diagnosis of infertility and should never feel shame or guilt for allowing medicine to aid in their struggle. It takes a tremendous amount of character and strength to face an in vitro cycle, and whether a couple is successful in their endeavors or not, I commend every infertile couple for chasing their baby dreams.

At one time, I too looked to the future and saw only darkness and disappointment. I felt the joy of life growing inside me only to have it stolen much too soon. I struggled, I stumbled and many times I fell. But through it all, I kept moving forward, searching for hope. In vitro fertilization gave me hope. It gave me opportunity. But most importantly, it gave me Nicholas. A sweet little boy who is a part of me and a part of Jeff and a testament to the love we have for each other. This is the beauty of alphabet blessings.

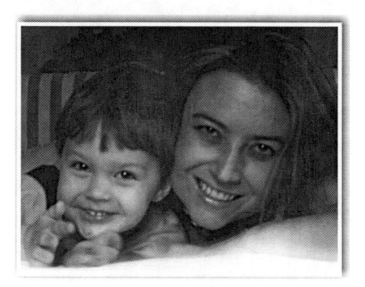

Author Bio

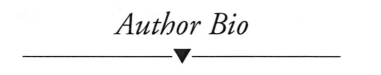

After choosing to walk away from a career in clinical medicine, Jenifer Cotter currently focuses her energy on raising her son and expressing herself as a writer and artist. She graduated cum laude with a Bachelor of Arts in biology and a Bachelor of Arts in pre-med, and earned her degree as a Doctor of Osteopathic Medicine (D.O.) at the Chicago College of Osteopathic Medicine. Jenifer made the difficult decision to leave medicine after losing her first pregnancy and beginning her painful battle with infertility.

Jenifer's IVF success story Web site sparked her creative side and began her support endeavors at a time when her life had been consumed by pain and sadness for her inability to conceive. Following the birth of her son, she branched into managing an infertility/IVF support group and began writing articles geared towards education on the subjects of infertility and assisted reproductive technologies. Countless interactions over a five year period with infertile couples who felt lost and afraid inspired Jenifer to increase her writing efforts with the hope of reaching more couples.

Jenifer holds true to her training as a physician by offering much of herself in order to help others. Her unique appreciation of motherhood following infertility, her holistic medical background and her artistic talents, lend a very personal and honest touch to her writing and infertility support endeavors.

DAY	LUPRON	DRUG	DOSE	EVENT	DOXY	ASA	PROG
1							
2							
3	0.5 mg					1	
4	0.5 mg					1	
5	0.5 mg					1	
6	0.5 mg					1	
7	0.5 mg					1	
8	0.5 mg					1	
9	0.5 mg					1	
10	0.5 mg					1	
11	0.5 mg					1	
12	0.5 mg					1	
13	0.5 mg					1	
14	0.5 mg					1	
15		Gonal-F	4amps	menses		1	
16		Gonal-F	4amps			1	
17		Gonal-F	4amps			1	
18		Gonal-F	4amps			1	
19		Gonal-F	4amps			1	
20		Gonal-F	4amps			1	
21		Gonal-F	4amps			1	
22		Gonal-F	4amps			1	
23		Gonal-F	4amps			1	
24		Gonal-F	4amps			1	
25		Gonal-F	4amps			1	
26				hCG	1	1	
27					1+1	1	
28				ER	1	1	1 sup
29						1	1 sup
30						1	1 sup
31						1	1 sup
32						1	1 sup
33						1	1 sup
34						1	1 sup
35						1	1 sup
36						1	1 sup
37						1	1 sup
38						1	1 sup
39						1	1 sup
40						1	1 sup
41				Spotting		1	1 sup
42				Bleed		1	1+1
43				Spotting		1	1+1
44				Bleed		1	PIO
51							1+1
57							1+1
66							1 sup

Sup = Crinone vaginal suppository, PIO = progesterone in oil (50mg twice a day), ASA = aspirin

E2	LH	P4	hCG	Follicle size	U/S	Endometrium	DAY
							1
							2
		6.8					3
							4
							5
							6
							7
							8
							9
							10
							11
							12
							13
							14
68	4			<5mm		13.5mm	15
							16
							17
							18
73	<1			6.9-7.7mm		6.2mm	19
							20
							21
243	<1			8.2-11.1mm		10.2mm	22
							23
479	1			11.1-12.6mm		11.4mm	24
							25
1449	3			14.9-17.7mm		12.3mm	26
							27
							28
							29
							30
							31
							32
							33
							34
							35
							36
							37
							38
							39
							40
							41
							42
							43
							44
					Sac		51
					FHT		57
					FHT		66

Follicle size = right & left ovary, Sac = gestational sac, FHT = fetal heart tones/ heartbeat

Alphabet Soup

▼

One of the most daunting tasks as an infertility couples is learning the lingo and acronyms that surround infertility, treatments, procedures, bulletin boards and online support groups. IVFers have developed their own way of discussing very complex issues in order to keep them more personal and add a human touch.

You may hear IVFers refer to the alphabet soup of assisted reproductive technologies. Alphabet soup refers to the numerous acronyms used when discussing infertility and ART. The following list is a collection of acronyms that will help you communicate more effectively with your RE and support group members. Many support groups will develop their own acronyms, so it is always a good idea to lurk for a few days before posting if you aren't comfortable with the shorthand they use.

2WW—Two-week wait

AH—Assisted hatching

AF—Aunt Flo

AMA—Advanced maternal age or antimicrosomal antibodies or American Medical Association

APA—Antiphospholipid antibodies

APLS—Antiphospholipid antibody syndrome

ARD—Adhesion related disorder

ART—Assisted reproductive technologies

ASA—Aspirin

ATA—Antithyroglobulin antibody

AZH—Assisted hatching

BA—Baby aspirin

Baby dust—Way to send good luck to someone TTC

BB—Bulletin board

BBT—Basal body temperature

BCP—Birth control pills

BD—Baby dance (sexual intercourse)

BFN—Big fat negative (negative pregnancy test)

BFP—Big fat positive (positive pregnancy test)

BFTA—Big fat try again (for those who feel BFN is too depressing)

BIL—Brother-in-law

BM—Birth mom, used when discussing adoption

BMS—Baby-making sex

BRB—Be right back or bright red blood/bleeding

BT—Blastocyst transfer

BTDT—Been there, done that

BTW—By the way

B/W, BW—Blood work

BX—Biopsy

CB—Cycle buddy

CCCT/CCT—Clomiphine citrate challenge test/Clomid challenge test

CD—Cycle day

CM—Cervical mucus

CMV—Cytomegalovirus

D&C—Dilation & curettage

DD—Dear daughter

DE—Donor egg

DES—Diethylstilbestrol

DH—Dear husband

DI—Donor insemination

DIL—Daughter-in-law

DOR—Decreased ovarian reserve

Dpo/DPO—Days post ovulation

Dpr/DPR—Days post retrieval

Dpt/DPT—Days post-transfer. An example is 10dp5dt, meaning 10 days post a 5 day transfer. IVF patients track their two week wait and beta tests this way.

DS—Dear son or donor sperm

dt—Day transfer. A 3dt means the embryos were transferred back 3 days after fertilization. A 5dt means the embryos were transferred 5 days after fertilization.

DW—Dear wife

Dx—Diagnosis

E2—Estradiol
ED—Egg donor
Endo—Endometriosis
ER—Egg retrieval
ET—Embryo transfer
FAQ—Frequently asked questions
FET—Frozen embryo transfer
FIL—Father-in-law
Follies—Follicles
FSH—Follicle-stimulating hormone
GAST—Gonadotropin-releasing hormone agonist (GnRHa) stimulation test
GES/GESS—Graduated embryo score/graduated embryo scoring system
GIFT—Gamete intrafallopian transfer
GnRH—Gonadotropin-releasing hormone
GnRHa—Gonadotropin-releasing hormone agonist
GS—Gestational surrogate
HB/hb—heartbeat
hCG—Human chorionic gonadotropin
HOM—High order multiples (triplets, quadruplets, etc.)
HPT—Home pregnancy test

HSC—Hysteroscopy
HSG—Hysterosalpingogram
HTH—Hope this/that helps
ICSI—Intracytoplasmic sperm injection
IF—Infertility
IMHO—In my humble opinion
IMO—In my opinion
IUI—Intrauterine insemination
IN—Intranasal
IVF—In vitro fertilization
IVFer—Person or couple undergoing in vitro to conceive
IVIg—Intravenous immunoglobin
JK—Just kidding
Lap—Laparoscopic surgery
LH—Luteinizing hormone
LMAO—Laugh my ass off
LMP—Last menstrual period
LOL—Laugh out loud
LPD—Luteal phase defect
LSC—Low sperm count
MC—Miscarriage
MCF—Microflare protocol
MESA—Microepididymal sperm aspiration, microsurgical epididymal sperm aspiration
MF—Male factor

MIL—Mother-in-law

MS—Morning sickness

NT—No text (message board when title or subject is only text)

"O"—Most often refers to ovulation rather than orgasm

OHSS—Ovarian hyperstimulation syndrome

OPK—Ovulation predictor kit

OTC—Over the counter

P4—Progesterone

PCOS—Polycystic ovarian syndrome

PCT—Post-coital test

PESA—Percutaneous epididymal sperm aspiration

PG—Pregnant, pregnancy

PGD—Pre-implantation genetic diagnosis

PID—Pelvic inflammatory disease

PIH—Pregnancy-induced hypertension

PIO—Progesterone in oil

PMS—Premenstrual syndrome

POAS—Pee on a stick

POF—Premature ovarian failure

PUPO—Pregnant until proven otherwise

RE—Reproductive endocrinologist

ROTF—Rolling on the floor

RPL—Recurrent pregnancy loss

RX—Prescription

SA—Semen analysis

SAHD—Stay-at-home dad

SAHM—Stay-at-home mom

SD—Sperm donor

SIL—Sister-in-law

SO—Significant other

SR—Selective reduction

S/S, S&S—Signs and symptoms

STI—Sexually transmitted infection

STD—Sexually transmitted disease

subQ/SQ—Subcutaneous

Sx/SX—Surgery

TESE—Transepididymal sperm aspiration

TET—Tubal embryo transfer

TFNA—Testicular fine needle aspiration

TMET—Transmyometrial embryo transfer

TMI—Too much information

TTC—Trying to conceive

TX—Treatment

UGET—Ultrasound guided embryo transfer

U/S—Ultrasound

UTI—Urinary tract infection

WAHD—Work-at-home dad

WAHM—Work-at-home mom

ZIFT—Zygote intrafallopian transfer

Learn the Lingo

▼

When you pursue parenthood with the help of in vitro fertilization or frozen embryo transfer, you suddenly find yourself buried under technical terminology. This section contains a list of common terms, medications and procedures to help you better understand the content of this book, Web sites and their newsletters.

Adhesions—Normal healing process the body undergoes to repair damaged or cut tissue or cells. Abnormal or excessive formation of adhesions can lead to infertility issues. Fibrous tissue resulting from an inflammatory response.

Adhesion related disorder—The normal response of the peritoneal lining (the thin layer of cells along the abdominal and pelvic cavities) is to produce a material that is reabsorbed and allows healing to occur without scar formation. An abnormal response of the peritoneal lining is to produce a material that is not absorbed by the body, causing an inflammatory reaction. Adhesion related disorder (ARD) is a condition in which adhesions have formed such that there is chronic pain and disruption of the daily activities of living. In women, ARD can cause or contribute to infertility.

Acupuncture—Part of traditional Chinese medicine, the application of needles over specific points (located on meridians) to stimulate chi, to balance excess or deficient energies.

Agglutination—Adhesion of parts, clumping.

Amps—Unit of measurement.

Anembryonic gestation—Visible embryo never develops within gestational sac.

Aneuploidy—Higher or lower chromosome number than normal (i.e. Down syndrome)

Antagon—Gonadotropin-releasing hormone agonist (GnRHa) medication that is given subcutaneously and blocks the premature release of luteinizing hormone (LH) prior to ovulation.

Antimicrosomal antibodies (AMA)—Example of antithyroid antibody, antibody directed against thyroid gland.

Antiphospholipid antibodies (APA)—Antibodies directed against phospholipids (fats that contain phosphorous), found in antiphospholipid antibody syndrome.

Antiphospholipid antibody syndrome (APLS)—An immune disorder characterized by the presence of abnormal antibodies in the blood associated with abnormal blood clotting, migraine headaches, low platelet counts and recurrent pregnancy loss.

Antithyroglobulin antibody (ATA)—Nonspecific autoantibodies that are frequently associated with endometriosis and pelvic adhesions.

Antral follicle count—Transvaginal ultrasound evaluation of the number of antral follicles present in the ovaries. The antral follicle count predicts the ovarian response to gonadotropin stimulation.

Aspermia—Condition in which there is no ejaculate.

Aspirate—To withdraw from.

Assisted hatching (AZH/AH)—The embryo must break out of its shell (hatch) before attaching itself to the uterine wall. Assisted hatching involves creating a small opening in the outer shell (either chemically or mechanically) to aid in attachment. Most often, an acidified Tyrode's solution is used to thin the zona pellucida. Assisted hatching can increase implantation significantly in eggs otherwise unlikely to fertilize unassisted. This is more commonly done in older women or those who have had previously unsuccessful IVF protocols.

Assisted reproductive technologies (ART)—Encompasses those techniques and technologies used to assist with conception.

Asthenzoospermia—Condition in which there is less than 50 percent spermatozoa with forward progression.

Atresia—Death of a cell.

Azoospermia—This means the man's sperm count is zero. He may still be producing sperm, but they cannot get out of the testes. No spermatozoa in ejaculate.

Beta—Quantitative blood test that measures the level of hCG circulating in a woman's blood.

Blastocele—Fluid-filled pocket of the blastocyst.

Blastocyst—Multi-celled stage at which implantation is possible.

Blastocyst transfer—Done 5-6 days after egg retrieval. More cell divisions have occurred and the quality is more discernible.

Blighted ovum—Development of normal looking gestational sac WITHOUT an embryo present (anembryonic gestation); usually occurs following embryonic death with continued trophoblast development. Empty sac contains no distinguishing structures within it.

Bravelle—Injectable gonadotropin used in stimulation stage of IVF cycle.

Braxton Hicks contractions—Commonly referred to as false labor, irregular contractions of the uterus during pregnancy.

Catheter—Thin tube of varying lengths and sizes.

Cervical canal—Canal which runs through the center of the cervix, connecting the vaginal vault on one side to the uterine cavity on the other side.

Cervical mucus (CM)—The mucus within the cervical canal. This mucus changes consistency during the different phases of the menstrual cycle. Women trying to conceive will often test their mucus to time sexual intercourse in order to increase their chances of conception.

Cervical os—The small opening within the center of the cervix which allows the sperm to enter the uterus.

Chemical pregnancy—Term used when there is a positive hCG level but no embryologic growth (i.e., a +HPT, but nothing seen on ultrasound).

Cilia—Small, hair-like projections that line the inside of the Fallopian tube and aid in the movement of the egg and sperm.

Clomid—Brand-name oral medication used to induce ovulation.

Clomiphene citrate—Generic name for Clomid and Serophene. Used to induce ovulation.

Clomiphene citrate challenge test (CCCT)—Also called Clomid challenge test, after receiving specific, timed doses of clomiphene citrate, blood levels of FSH and E2 are measured on Day 3 or Day 10 of the menstrual cycle to determine ovarian reserve. An elevated FSH level on Day 10 points to poor ovarian reserve.

Coasting—Withdrawal of exogenous gonadotropins (stimulation medications) in midst of IVF cycle until serum E2 level decreases.

Corpus luteum—Granulated mass in the ovary that is formed from the follicle once the egg has been released. It secretes progesterone. Remains for several months if pregnancy occurs or degenerates if no pregnancy occurs.

Corpus luteum cyst—Fluid-filled sac within ovary that may rupture about the time of menstruation and may take up to three months to disappear entirely.

Crinone—Medication which contains micronized progesterone, a vaginal suppository thought to help support early pregnancy.

Crowning—Point of delivery when the top of the baby's head pushes out.

Cryopreservation—The freezing of viable embryos, eggs or sperm to be used for in vitro or frozen embryo transfer.

Cycle—Although typically this refers to the menstrual cycle, in this book the term cycle most often refers to an in vitro fertilization cycle, which involves controlled ovarian hyperstimulation followed by egg retrieval, fertilization and embryo transfer. Cycles may or may not include initial down regulation (suppression).

Cycle Buddy—Support group terminology denoting those members who are cycling at the same time and chat about their cycles as they progress through the stages.

Cytomegalovirus (CMV)—Cytomegalovirus is a member of the herpes virus group and is spread through urine, saliva, semen, blood, tears and breast milk. Often asymptomatic, this virus usually remains dormant after the initial infection resolves. Produces no long-term health concerns except for the transmission to babies at time of delivery, children, and others with compromised immune systems.

Cytoplasm—Substance of the cell outside of the nucleus.

Decreased ovarian reserve (DOR)—Condition character-ized by diminished quantity and quality of eggs, diagnosed via Clomid challenge test, ovarian volume assessment, and/or antral follicle count.

Diethylstilbestrol (DES)—Synthetic estrogen used until the early 70's, when it was found to cause significant birth defects. Daughters of these women are at increased risk for certain cancers and infertility.

Dilation and curettage (D&C)—Procedure done to remove products of conception following a miscarriage or done to remove built-up endometrium.

Distal tubal occlusion—A blockage of the Fallopian tube that occurs distal to the uterine junction (i.e. at the end of the tube away from the uterus/closest to the ovary). Causes can include PID, infections near the pelvis such as appendicitis, infections of the ovary, lower abdominal or pelvic surgery, and endometriosis. The damage inflicted may result in occlusion of the distal end of the tube (the end closest to the ovary); destruction of the cilia and/or fimbria; adhesions outside the tube, which distort the normal course of the tube; and dilation of the tube with the presence of inflammatory fluid (hydrosalpinx).

Donor egg (DE)—Refers to the egg that has been donated.

Donor insemination (DI)—Procedure of insemination using donated sperm.

Donor sperm (DS)—Refers to the sperm that has been donated.

Down regulation—Suppression of the woman's ovaries that drops estrogen levels and prevents ovulation.

Doxycycline—Broad spectrum antibiotic used during an in vitro cycle to protect against infection following egg retrieval.

Eclampsia—Final phase of preeclampsia, occurrence of seizures in addition to swelling, high blood pressure, and protein in the urine.

Ectopic—A pregnancy occurring outside the uterus, often in the Fallopian tube.

Egg—Oocyte, produced by the woman's ovaries and fertilized by the man's sperm.

Egg donor—Refers to the individual who has donated eggs to another couple.

Egg retrieval (ER)—Process of inserting needle into ovarian follicles to withdraw eggs. Also a general term for the retrieval phase of an IVF cycle.

Embies—Endearing name given to our embryos.

Embryo—Next stage of development after the zygote.

Embryologist—A scientist who studies the formation, early development, and growth of living organisms.

Embryo transfer (ET)—Procedure done 2-5 days after retrieval. A catheter inserted through the cervix allows placement of the embryo(s) inside the uterus. Also a general term for the transfer phase of an IVF cycle.

Endometrial biopsy—Test performed to determine if the lining of the uterus is maturing at the proper rate to permit a fertilized egg to implant and grow. It is performed on the twelfth luteal day, or two days before an expected menses. During the luteal phase, the lining of the uterus undergoes specific cell changes. Microscopic examination of a small sample of the uterus lining tells the RE if the woman's endometrium is changing properly. A thin plastic catheter is inserted through the cervix into the uterus, and a small piece of endometrial tissue is removed. An endometrial biopsy only takes a few minutes, but it can cause cramping.

Endometrium—Innermost layer that lines the uterine cavity.

Endometrial lining—Tissue that lines the uterus. This tissue is referred to as the endometrial lining and thickens in preparation for implantation of an embryo. If implantation does not occur, the lining is shed with the woman's period.

Endometriosis (Endo)—Disease process that occurs when tissue that normally lines the uterine cavity implants and grows outside the uterus. These endometrial foci (areas of endometrial tissue) most often occur on or near the reproductive organs, especially around the Fallopian tubes. As with the uterine endometrial tissue, the endometrial foci respond to ovarian hormones.

Epididymis—Small collecting tubules located next to the testes.

Episiotomy—Surgical cut during labor to enlarge vaginal opening prior to delivery of the baby's head.

Estradiol (E2)—Precursor of estrogen. Most of IVFers interchange estrogen and estradiol when discussing their cycles. This is monitored during an in vitro cycle with blood tests.

Estrogen—Hormone responsible for producing an environment suitable for fertilization, implantation, and nutrition of the early embryo.

Evil pee stick—Term used by infertility couples when discussing a home pregnancy test.

Exogenous—Originating externally, derived from outside of the body.

Fallopian tube—A muscular structure approximately 10 cm long that functions as a passageway between the ovary and uterus. The diameter of the Fallopian tube is quite small where it joins the uterus, and then slowly increases toward the end where the fimbria are located. These fimbria are responsible for drawing the newly released, mature egg into the Fallopian tube, where it will continue to move towards the uterus.

Both tubes are capable of highly coordinated movement. This is possible due to the millions of cilia which line the tube itself. These cilia are responsible for movement of the eggs, sperm, and embryos. The Fallopian tube lining is capable of producing a fluid, which provides nutrition to the egg, and aids the sperm in penetrating the egg at fertilization.

Fertilization—A process whereby the sperm penetrates the egg and genetic material is combined from both the sperm and the egg; typically occurs in Fallopian tube with unassisted conception.

Fibroid—Benign (non-cancerous) tumor/growth of uterine wall.

Fimbria—Finger-like projections located on the end of the Fallopian tube closest to the ovary.

Follicle—Fluid-filled structure within ovary comprised of oocyte and the surrounding cell layer.

Follicle-stimulating hormone (FSH)—A gonadotropin hormone that is secreted by the anterior pituitary and stimulates the growth and maturation of ovarian follicles in females. This hormone is critical for sperm production in males.

Follicular cyst—Most common type of ovarian cyst that results from the growth of a follicle. In some menstrual cycles, the follicle grows larger than normal and fails to rupture, thus not releasing the egg. Typically, a follicular cyst resolves with simple observation over the course of days to months.

Follicular phase—Occurs between days one to thirteen or fourteen of menstrual cycle. Phase during which follicles grow and endometrium thickens.

Follistim—Injectable gonadotropin used in stimulation stage of IVF cycle.

Fragmentation—Cytoplasm of cell is ejected during normal cell division, little to no fragmentation is considered normal.

Fresh cycle—Refers to in vitro fertilization cycle which uses controlled hyperstimulation of the ovaries to produce eggs that are then fertilized. The resulting embryos are transferred back to the uterus in the hopes of achieving pregnancy.

Frosties—Endearing name given to frozen embryos.

Frozen embryo transfer (FET)—Embryos frozen from a fresh IVF cycle are thawed and then transferred into the uterus.

Functional cyst—Fluid-filled sac within the ovary that is part of the normal process of menstruation. Functional cysts can form during the suppression phase.

Gamete intrafallopian transfer (GIFT)—Three to four *unfertilized* eggs are mixed with sperm and a small amount of media, which is then transferred into the tube. Fertilization in the tube and migration into the uterus occurs as with unassisted conception.

Gestation—Time period from conception to delivery.

Gestational carrier—Woman who carries another couple's embryo/child for the term of the pregnancy.

Gestational sac—Small amniotic cavity in which the embryo will eventually develop, first detectable marker of potential pregnancy on ultrasound.

Gestational surrogate—See gestational carrier.

Gonadotropin—Stimulating hormone secreted by the pituitary gland. In women, this includes both follicle-stimulating hormone (FSH) and luteinizing hormone (LH). Also used when discussing urinary-derived FSH and/or LH, and recombinant DNA-derived FSH and LH.

Gonadotropin-releasing hormone (GnRH)—Originates from hypothalamus; when released, influences production of gonadotropin by pituitary gland. In an IVF cycle, this hormone stimulates the ovaries. GnRH regulates FSH and LH.

Gonadotropin-releasing hormone agonist (GnRHa)—Class of drugs used during an IVF cycle to suppress production of estrogen by ovaries.

Gonadotropin-releasing hormone agonist stimulation test (GAST)—Lupron is administered with measurement of serum E2 levels on cycle Day 2 and Day 3. Typically, the better the rise in the E2 level, the better the pregnancy rate.

Gonal-F—Recombinant gonadotropin used in stimulation stage of IVF cycle.

Graduate embryo score (GES)—System of grading Day 3 embryos to determine their likelihood of developing into blastocysts. Score is given out of 100 points, with those embryos scoring higher more likely to progress to the blastocyst stage.

Growth medium—Solution that promotes growth and development of the embryo in the laboratory setting.

Heterotopic pregnancy—Combined pregnancy. There are several forms of pregnancy: intrauterine, ectopic, false, intra-abdominal, and so on. If a woman has two types of pregnancy at the same time, i.e., intrauterine and ectopic, it is referred to as heterotopic.

High responder—Denotes woman you has an exaggerated response to gonadotropins (stimulation medications), with production of a greater number of eggs and a significantly elevated E2 level.

Hippocratic Oath—Oath taken by physicians that pertains to the ethical practice of medicine.

Home pregnancy test (HPT)—A home pregnancy test measures the hormone called human chorionic gonadotropin (hCG) to determine whether a woman is pregnant. A HPT determines if hCG is present in the urine. Different home pregnancy tests have different minimum levels of hCG they are able to detect (the test's sensitivity). This is a qualitative test, meaning it only tells if hCG is present, not the actual amount present.

Human chorionic gonadotropin (hCG)—Hormone produced by the embryo soon after conception and later by the placenta. This hormone level continues to rise during a normal pregnancy. Pregnancy tests detect these levels.

hCG level—Refers to the amount of human chorionic gonadotropin within the body. The hCG level is normally zero. The level increases by doubling every two to three days in early pregnancy.

hCG trigger—Injection of human chorionic gonadotropin which promotes final maturation of developing eggs.

Humegon—Human menopausal gonadotropin used in the stimulation stage of IVF cycle.

Hydrosalpinx—Condition that involves dilation of the Fallopian tube and the presence of inflammatory fluid within the tube.

Hysterosalpingogram—This procedure looks at both the uterus and the Fallopian tubes. A catheter is placed within the cervical canal and held in place by a small inflatable balloon, located at the catheter tip. A contrast dye is then injected through the catheter as X-rays are taken. The contrast fills the uterine cavity and then spills out through the Fallopian tubes on either side. No spillage occurs if the Fallopian tubes are completely blocked. Filling of the uterine cavity appears uneven in cases of uterine fibroids or polyps located within the uterus. Decreased or slowed spillage from the Fallopian tubes may indicate a partial blockage, although it does not necessarily indicate a blockage from within the tube itself, as with the case of adhesions. Some women experience only minimal discomfort with this procedure while other women, usually those with severe or complete blockage of the tube(s), may have significant pain. The dye that spills out of the Fallopian tubes or that remains within the uterine cavity is eventually absorbed by the body.

Hysteroscopy—This procedure uses fiberoptic technology, allowing the physician to visualize the uterine cavity directly. A small fiberoptic telescope is inserted into the uterine cavity through the cervical canal. Either gas or fluid may be infused into the uterine cavity in order to open the cavity to better visualize it. Many women experience only mild discomfort due to the infusion of the fluid or gas into the cavity.

Hysterosonogram—This is an ultrasound of the uterus. Most often, a catheter is placed within the cervical canal or uterine cavity and held in place by a small inflatable balloon found at the tip. Ultrasound is then used to visualize the uterus while fluid is injected through the catheter. The fluid may either be water, saline (salt water), or other fluids specifically intended for use with ultrasound imaging. Most women experience no or minimal discomfort with this procedure.

Immune factor infertility—Dysfunction of the immune system that interferes with the normal process of reproduction.

Implantation—Process whereby a fertilized egg attaches to the uterine lining.

Implantation bleeding or spotting—The slight discharge of blood that occurs following implantation similar to the spotting of a woman's period.

Infertility (IF)—The diminished ability or the inability to conceive and/or maintain a pregnancy to term. Infertility is also defined in specific terms as the failure to conceive after twelve months of regular intercourse without contraception, or after six months, if the woman is thirty-five years of age or older.

Inner cell mass—Component of a blastocyst, this will eventually form the embryo.

Intracytoplasmic sperm injection (ICSI)—A single isolated sperm is drawn up into a specially designed pipette. The pipette is inserted into the egg's center (the cytoplasm) and the sperm is released. This fertilization technique is used in couples with severe male factor.

Intramuscular (IM)—Injection into the muscle.

Intranasal—Administration within the nose, often sniffed.

Intrauterine insemination (IUI)—Sperm is placed within the uterine cavity at the time of ovulation.

Intravenous (IV)—Injection directly into the vein.

In vitro fertilization (IVF)—Form of ART where fertilization occurs in a special medium in a laboratory setting and then resulting embryo(s) are placed back into uterus.

Lupron—Gonadotropin-releasing hormone agonist, injectable, used in suppression stage of IVF cycle.

Lurker—Refers to member of an online support group/bulletin or message board who reads messages but does not actively participate in discussions.

Luteal phase—Phase of menstrual cycle when fertilization and implantation occur resulting in pregnancy. If fertilization or implantation does not occur, the woman will have her menses.

Luteal phase defect (LPD)—In this situation, cells of the endometrial lining do not correspond to the menstrual cycle days. Believed either to be due to lack of sufficient progesterone secretion by the corpus luteum, or failure of the endometrium to respond to ovarian steroids, making the endometrium insufficient to support implantation. Often diagnosed when the luteal phase of a woman's menstrual cycle is shorter than ten days.

Luteinizing hormone (LH)—Hormone which stimulates the secretion of testosterone from the testes and stimulates the ovary to secret testosterone which is then converted to estrogen. A burst of luteinizing hormone induces ovulation. LH is required for the corpus luteum to continue developing and functioning.

Lymphocyte—Small white blood cell involved in the body's defense mechanism.

Male factor infertility—This diagnosis is given when there is a problem with the man's sperm that causes or contributes to infertility. May be due to shape (morphology), quantity (concentration), or movement (motility). About 30 percent of infertility cases are due to male factor issues.

Microepididymal sperm aspiration (MESA)—A sperm retrieval procedure. Sperm is aspirated directly from the epididymis, used with ICSI.

Micromanipulation techniques—Includes the techniques of intracytoplasmic sperm injection, sub-zonal sperm insertion, partial zona dissection and assisted hatching.

Mitosis—Type of cell division human cells undergo to form an embryo.

Mock transfer—The procedure of placing a catheter through the cervical canal into the uterus without actually transferring any embryos.

Morula—Stage of development where 16-32 cells are present.

Newbie—Refers to a person who has just been diagnosed with infertility or is about to undergo their first in vitro cycle, typically used on online message boards.

Nubain—Narcotic pain reliever.

Oligospermia—The man's sperm count is sub-fertile, concentration is less than 20 million/ml.

Oocyte—An egg.

Ovarian cyst—Fluid-filled sac within the ovary. Any ovarian follicle that is larger than about 2 cm is termed an ovarian cyst. Types of cysts include follicular, corpus luteum and Graafian cyst. Other cysts are pathological, such as those found in polycystic ovary syndrome or those associated with tumors.

Ovarian hyperstimulation syndrome (OHSS)—A medical complication that may occur after gonadotropin use, such as with IVF. In its severe form, OHSS is characterized by ovarian enlargement and a build-up of fluid in the abdomen (ascites), chest cavity (pleural effusion), or around the heart (pericardial effusion). It affects blood electrolytes, liver and kidney function, and puts the patient at greater risk for blood clots. Patients may experience abdominal discomfort, nausea, vomiting, weight gain, decreased urine production, shortness of breath, difficulty breathing, or pelvic pain. If you experience these or have any concerns always contact your physician immediately. **Complications of OHSS can be FATAL.**

Ovarian reserve—Refers to the number of eggs (supply of eggs) and the ability of the ovaries to release mature eggs capable of fertilization; this decreases naturally with age. Ovarian reserve is closely associated with reproductive potential.

Ovarian torsion—Twisting of the ovary leading to extreme lower abdominal pain.

Ovulation—Release of a mature egg, ready for fertilization.

Ovulatory phase—Phase of menstrual cycle during which ovulation occurs.

PercBiopsy—Percutaneous (through the skin) biopsy of the testis done under local anesthesia.

Percutaneous epididymal sperm aspiration (PESA)—A sperm retrieval procedure. Sperm is aspirated directly from the epididymis; used with ICSI; can be done under local or general anesthesia.

Pergonal—Human menopausal gonadotropin used in stimulation stage of IVF cycle.

Perineum—In a woman, the area between the anus and vulva (labial opening to vagina).

Pfannenstiel incision—Transverse incision below the belly button and above the point where the pubic bones join, used during cesarean section delivery.

Pipette—Glass or transparent plastic tube used in measuring or transferring small amounts of liquid. Used with ICSI.

Pitocin induction—Use of the medication Pitocin to facilitate labor through increased uterine contractions.

Polycystic ovarian syndrome (PCOS)—Condition in which a hormonal imbalance affects ovulation. PCOS occurs in 5-10 percent of women aged twenty to forty, and includes such symptoms as acne, irregular menses, excessive hair growth and weight gain. There is a lack of ovulation and there are enlarged ovaries containing one or more abnormal cysts.

Polyp—Tissue mass that develops within a hollow organ, such as the colon or uterus.

Poor responder—Denotes woman who has a suboptimal response to gonadotropins (stimulation medications) during an IVF cycle, with few eggs produced and low E2 levels achieved.

Potency—Measure of a drug's activity within the body.

Preeclampsia—The presence of hypertension or pregnancy-induced hypertension, proteinuria (protein in urine), and edema (swelling), often referred to as toxemia of pregnancy. Preeclampsia which goes untreated, or does not respond to treatment, leads to eclampsia which can be fatal to both mother and baby.

Pregnancy-induced hypertension (PIH)—Hypertension that occurs during pregnancy, often requiring medication. Some risk factors for PIH include first pregnancy, multiple gestations (twins, triplets, etc.), and family history.

Pregnyl—Injectable medication containing hormone hCG. Used primarily to trigger ovulation.

Pre-implantation genetic diagnosis (PGD)—Pre-implantation genetic diagnosis is testing done to check for genetic abnormalities in an embryo, typically at the 4-8 cell stage prior to transferring it back to the woman. Detects chromosomal composition and presence or absence of specific genes.

Premature ovarian failure (POF)—Also called early menopause, the ovaries of an otherwise healthy woman stop functioning before naturally reaching menopause.

Preparation phase—Phase of an IVF cycle which includes pre-cycle testing and any procedures to prepare the body for IVF and pregnancy.

Profasi—Injectable medication containing hormone hCG. Used primarily to trigger ovulation.

Progesterone—Steroid hormone normally produced by the corpus luteum after ovulation and by the placenta during pregnancy.

Proliferative phase—See follicular phase.

Proximal tubal occlusion—A blockage that occurs at the junction of the uterus and Fallopian tube. Causes can include spasm of the uterine wall (giving a temporary occlusion), small plugs of mucoid material, endometriosis and adhesions.

Reglan pump—Small pump which dispenses Reglan (anti-nausea medication) through a small catheter into the woman's body.

Reproductive endocrinologist (RE)—A subspecialist in obstetrics and gynecology who deals with reproductive endocrinology and infertility-related issues in women, and who has successfully completed a graduate education program at least thirty-six months in duration.

Repronex—Human menopausal gonadotropin used in stimulation stage of IVF cycle.

Secretory phase—See luteal phase.

Selective reduction—Procedure by which the number of developing fetuses is reduced in the first trimester of pregnancy, most often considered in pregnancies of triplets or higher order multiples.

Semen analysis—A test performed on a fresh specimen that looks at both quantity and quality of sperm. The quality of the sperm is further broken down into morphology (shape) and motility (movement).

Serophene—Brand name for clomiphene citrate, used to induce ovulation.

Sexually transmitted infection/disease (STI/STD)—Includes Chlamydia, gonorrhea, herpes, HPV, hepatitis, syphilis, trichomoniasis, CMV and HIV.

Sperm Donor (SD)—Refers to the individual who donates his sperm.

Spermatozoa—Sperm, responsible for fertilizing the egg, comprised of head, neck, middle piece, and tail with end piece.

Stenotic—Narrowing of an opening.

Stimulation phase—Phase of an IVF cycle that uses exogenous gonadotropins to induce formation of multiple, mature eggs that are then retrieved.

Subcutaneous—Just beneath the skin, as with an injection.

Suppression phase—Phase of an IVF cycle that uses gonadotropin-releasing hormone agonists (GnRHa) to down regulate the ovaries, thus preventing ovulation.

Synarel—Inhalation gonadotropin-releasing hormone agonist, used in suppression stage of IVF cycle.

Teratozoospermia—Condition in which less than 30 percent normal spermatozoa morphology is present.

Testicular biopsy—Under local or general anesthesia, a small opening in the testis is surgically created. A small sample of tissue is then taken.

Testicular fine needle aspiration (TFNA)—Under local anesthesia, the needle punctures through the skin into the testis to extract sperm.

Testicular sperm extraction (TESA)—Small samples of testicular tissue are obtained through needle biopsy. Sperm are dissected out of the tissue for use in ICSI.

Totsicles—Endearing name given to frozen embryos.

Transabdominal sonography—Ultrasound technique where the probe is placed on the outside of the abdomen.

Transmyometrial transfer (TMT)—For this procedure, a needle is inserted through the wall of the uterus in order to transfer embryos. Reasons for performing this procedure include cervical stenosis, acute angle of the cervical canal, "fragile" embryos, and multiple implantation failures.

Transvaginal sonography—Ultrasound technique that utilizes a small probe placed within the vagina. This technique allows better visualization of the reproductive organs and allows earlier visualization of a developing embryo.

Trigger shot—Injection of hCG given to set in motion the final maturation of the eggs. Same as hCG trigger.

Trophectoderm—Outer cell layer of a blastocyst that eventually develops into the placenta in a viable pregnancy.

Tubal factor infertility—Infertility due to disease or abnormality of the Fallopian tube. Accounts for 20 to 30 percent of infertility cases. Evaluation of the tubes is needed to determine the severity of disease. Factors influencing the severity include diameter of hydrosalpinx (if present), the number of fimbria present, the functionality of the fimbria, the presence of adhesions surrounding the tube and/or ovary, and the number of rugae (folds) present within the tube itself.

Tuboplasty—Surgical procedure to correct obstruction of Fallopian tube in order to achieve pregnancy.

Two week wait (2WW)—The days or weeks following embryo transfer. A pregnancy test is performed at the end of the two week wait.

Ultrasound—Imaging, also referred to as ultrasonography, which allows physicians and patients to view soft tissues and body cavities without using invasive techniques.

Unexplained infertility—Diagnosis of infertility that has a cause which cannot be explained through testing.

Uterine fundus—Anatomic region of the body of the uterus.

Uterine Receptivity—The window of uterine receptivity for embryo implantation is a relatively short period of time (a few days in humans) during the luteal phase of the menstrual cycle. This is the time during which an embryo is able to successfully adhere to/implant within the endometrial lining of the uterus.

Uterine septum—Abnormal structure within the uterus which divides the cavity.

Viable—Able to sustain life.

Veteran—Refers to a person who has cycled numerous times without success.

Yolk sac—First element seen in the gestational sac in early pregnancy; the thickening of its margin leads to development of the embryo.

Zona pellucida—The thin outer shell of the oocyte/egg.

Zygote—A fertilized egg.

Zygote intrafallopian transfer (ZIFT)—The eggs and sperm are collected and allowed to fertilize in a special medium in a laboratory setting. They are then transferred back to the woman's Fallopian tube, where they will, it is hoped, migrate into the uterus and implant.

Infertility Resources

▼

American Fertility Association
http://www.theafa.org

American Pregnancy Association
http://www.americanpregnancy.org

American Society of Reproductive Medicine
http://www.asrm.org

International Council on Infertility Information Dissemination
http://www.inciid.org

INCIID list of states mandating infertility coverage
http://www.inciid.org/article.php?cat=&id=275

Infertility Network
http://www.infertilitynetwork.org

Medline Plus Infertility Information Page
http://www.nlm.nih.gov/medlineplus/infertility.html

National Infertility Network Exchange
http://www.nine-infertility.org

Resolve
http://www.resolve.org

Society for Male Reproduction and Urology
http://www.smru.org

Endnotes

—————————▼—————————

1   Centers for Disease Control Reproductive Health, "2003 Assisted Reproductive Technology (ART) Report," http://www.cdc.gov/ ART/index.htm.

2   Chandra, A., et al, "Fertility, Family Planning, and Reproductive Health of U.S. Women: Data from the 2002 National Survey of Family Growth," National Center for Health Statistics, Vital Health Statistics, *PHS* 23d ser., 25 (2005).

3   Centers for Disease Control Reproductive Health, "2003 Assisted Reproductive Technology (ART) Report: Section 5—Trends in ART, 1996–2003," http://www.cdc.gov/ART/ART2003/section5. htm.

4   CM Verhaak, et al, "Stress and Marital Satisfaction Among Women Before and After Their First Cycle of In Vitro Fertilization and Intracytoplasmic Sperm Injection," *Fertility and Sterility* 76, no. 3 (September 2001):525-31.

5   Gregory E. Chow, et al, "Antral Follicle Count and Serum Follicle-Stimulating Hormone Levels to Assess Functional Ovarian Age," *Obstetrics and Gynecology* 104, (2004):801-804.

6   Chang MY, et al, "The Antral Follicle Count Predicts the Outcome of Pregnancy in a Controlled Ovarian Hyperstimulation/ Intrauterine Insemination Program," *Journal of Assisted Reproductive Genetics* 15, no.1 (1998):7-12.

7   Ilkka Y. Järvelä, et al, "Quantification of Ovarian Power Doppler Signal with Three-Dimensional Ultrasonography to Predict Response During In Vitro Fertilization," *Obstetrics and Gynecology* 102, (2003):816-822.

8   Gregory E. Chow.

9   Chang MY.

10   Ibid.

[11] Ilkka Y. Järvelä.

[12] L. Rrumbullaku, "Semen Analysis," Geneva Foundation for Medical Education and Research, http://www.gfmer.ch/Endo/PGC_network/Semen_analysis_rrumbullaku.htm.

[13] Ibid.

[14] O. Levinsohn-Tavor, et al, "Coasting—What is the Best Formula?," *Human Reproduction* 18, no.5 (May 2003):937-940

[15] Ibid.

[16] Robert N. Clarke, et al, "Relationship Between Psychological Stress and Semen Quality Among In-Vitro Fertilization Patients," *Human Reproduction* 14, no. 3 (March 1999):753-758.

[17] T. Timothy Smith, "IVF Timetable and Embryo Grading," Shared Journey, Your Path to Fertility, http://www.sharedjourney.com/articles/Time.html.

[18] Staff of Karande & Associates, S.C. for Fertility, "Embryo Cryopreservation: What Should You Consider?" *Hope* 26, no. 3 (summer 2004).

[19] Susan M. Adams, et al, "Endometrial Response to IVF Hormonal Manipulation Comparative Analysis of Menopausal, Down Regulated and Natural Cycles," *Reproductive Biology and Endocrinology* 2 (2004):21.

[20] Vicken Sepilian and Ellen Wood, "Ectopic Pregnancy," eMedicine, http://www.emedicine.com/med/topic3212.htm, October 2005

[21] Heather B. Clayton, et al, "Ectopic Pregnancy Risk with Assisted Reproductive Technology Procedures", Obstetrics and Gynecology 107, no. 3 (March 2006):595-604.

[22] Creighton University School of Medicine Diagnostic & Interventional Radiology Department, Early Ultrasound Findings of Pregnancy, Creighton University Medical Center, http://radiology.creighton.edu/pregnancy.htm.

[23] Ibid.

[24] Ibid.

[25] Ibid.

26 Elizabeth Puscheck and Archana Pradham, "First Trimester Pregnancy Loss," eMedicine, http://www.emedicine.com/med/topic3310.htm, June 2006

27 The American Pregnancy Association, "Preconception Nutrition," http://www.americanpregnancy.org/gettingpregnant/preconception nutrition.html.

28 Alice Domar, "Engaging Mind and Body in Overcoming Infertility," *Hope* 26, no.3 (summer 2004).

29 Mary Ann Emanuele and Nicholas Emanuele, "Alcohol & the Male Reproductive System," National Institute on Alcohol Abuse and Alcoholism, http://www.niaaa.nih.gov/publications/arh25-4/282-287.htm.

30 Philip Shihua Li, "Lifestyle and Dietary Recommendations for the Infertile Man," Cornell Institute Center for Male Reproductive Medicine and Microsurgery, http://www.maleinfertility.com.

31 Ibid.

32 Ejaz Hassan Khan, et al, "Long Term Effects of Opiate Addiction on Male Fertility", *Journal of Postgraduate Institute* 17, no. 2 (2003):226-230.

33 Philip Shihua Li, "Lifestyle and Dietary Recommendations for the Infertile Man," Cornell Institute Center for Male Reproductive Medicine and Microsurgery, http://www.maleinfertility.org/lifestyle.html.

34 ASRM Patient Fact Sheet, "Obese Women Weight and Fertility," (August 2001).

35 Tina Kold Jensen, et al, "Body Mass Index in Relation to Semen Quality and Reproductive Hormones Among 1,558 Danish Men", *Fertility and Sterility* 82, no. 4 (2004):863-870.

36 Philip Shihua Li, "Lifestyle and Dietary Recommendations for the Infertile Man," Cornell Institute Center for Male Reproductive Medicine and Microsurgery, http://www.maleinfertility.org/lifestyle.html.

37 Robert J. Stillman, "Fertility Supplements for Male Infertility," IntegraMed America, http://www.integramed.com/inmdweb/content/cons/conceptions/fertility-supplements.jsp.

38 Support group discussions with author and members under the care of acupuncturists and herbalists for elevated FSH, The Baby Chase IVF Support Group (accessed 2004)

39 Martin Bastuba, "Man's Health—Stay Healthy," MaleFertility.MD, http://www.male-infertility-treatments.com/stay_healthy.html.

40 Stanton Honig, "Preventive Medicine and Male Factor Infertility: Facts and Fiction," Resolve: The National Infertility Association, North East Region, http://www.resolvenyc.org/MaleFactor.htm.

41 Hiliary Klonoff-Cohen and Loki Natarajan, "The Concerns During ART (CART) Scale & and Pregnancy Outcomes", *Fertility and Sterility* 81 no. 4 (April 2004).

42 Hiliary Klonoff-Cohen, et al, "A Prospective Study of Stress Among Women Undergoing In Vitro Fertilization or Gamete Intrafallopian Transfer," *Fertility and Sterility* 76, no. 4 (October 2001):675-687.

43 Aniruddha Malpani and Anjali Malpani, "Stress and Infertility", Adoption—Information, International, Domestic, Child and Agency Adoptions, Stories and Laws, http://www.adoption.com

44 Ernest Hung Yu Ng, et al, "HMG is as Good as Recombinant Human FSH in Terms of Oocyte and Embryo Quality: A Prospective Randomized Trial," *Human Reproduction* 16, no.2 (February 2001):319-325.

45 Dianne Clapp, "Smoking and Fertility," Family Building 4, no.1 (autumn 2004):10.

46 Dianne Clapp, "Smoking and Fertility," *Family Building* 4, no. 1 (autumn 2004): 10.

47 Michael Soules, "Preserving Your Fertility," Resolve Online Chat, http://www.resolve.org, (accessed September 9, 2003)

48 Philip Shihua Li, "Factors Affecting Results of ICSI," Cornell Institute Center for Male Reproductive Medicine and Microsurgery, http://www.maleinfertility.com/new-icsi.html

49 American Society for Reproductive Medicine, "Age and Fertility," Patient Fact Sheet (2003).

50 Jenkins JM, "The Influence, Development and Management of Functional Ovarian Cysts During IVF Cycles," *Human Reproduction* 1, no. 2, 11 Natl Suppl (1996):132-136.

51 Ernest Hung Yu Ng.

52 Millenova Immunology Laboratories, "Antithyroid (Thyroglobulin and Microsomal) Antibodies (ATA): Testing at Millenova Immunology Laboratories," http://www.millenova.com/tests/ata.asp.

53 Thyroid Foundation of Canada, "Thyroid Disease, Pregnancy and Fertility," http://www.thyroid.ca/Guides/HG08.html#Infertility

54 Ernest Hung Yu Ng.

55 ASRM patient fact sheet, "Prediction of Fertility Potential (Ovarian Reserve) in Women," (2005).

56 Chang MY, et al.

57 Sher Institutes for Reproductive Health, "SIRM: The Role of Antiphospholipid Antibodies (APA), Natural Killer (NK) Cells and Endometrial Cytokines in Immunologic Implantation Failure," http://www.haveababy.com/infert/implantfail.asp.

58 Millenova Immunology Laboratories, "Antiphospholipid Antibodies Panel (APA): Testing at Millenova Immunology Laboratories," http://www.millenova.com/tests/apa.asp.

59 Philip Shihua Li, "Factors Affecting Results of ICSI," Cornell Institute Center for Male Reproductive Medicine and Microsurgery, http://www.maleinfertility.com/new-icsi.html

60 Paul P.G., "Tubal Surgery in the Era of ART," Dr. Paul P.G. Gynecological Endoscopic Surgeon, http://www.paulpg.com/pdfs/tubularsurgery_ieoa.pdf.

61 D.A. Grainger, et al, "Racial Disparity in Clinical Outcomes from Women Using ART: Analysis of 80,196 ART Cycles from the SART Database 1999–2000," *Fertility and Sterility* 82, suppl 2 (September 2004):S37-S38.

62 Ernest Hung Yu Ng.

63 P. Lesney, et al, "Ultrasound Evaluation of the Uterine Zonal Anatomy During In Vitro Fertilization and Embryo Transfer," *Human Reproduction* 14, no. 6 (June 1999):593-1598.

64   Ernest Hung Yu Ng.

65   Ibid.

66   Rajneesh S. Mathur, et al, "Distinction Between Early and Late Ovarian Hyperstimulation Syndrome," *Fertility and Sterility* 73, no. 5 (May 2000):901-907.

67   Francisco Fábregues, et al, "Oocyte Quality in Patients with Severe Ovarian Hyperstimulation Syndrome: A Self-Controlled Clinical Study," *Fertility and Sterility* 82, no.4 (October 2004): 827-833.

Index

978-0-595-39524-8
0-595-39524-4